AFRICAN AMERICAN MEDICINE IN WASHINGTON, D.C.

AFRICAN AMERICAN MEDICINE IN WASHINGTON, D.C.

Healing the Capital During the Civil War Era

HEATHER BUTTS, JD, MPH, MA

Foreword by Dr. Hugh Florenz Butts, MD

THE History PRESS

Published by The History Press
Charleston, SC 29403
www.historypress.net

Cover: An operating room circa 1900 at the Frederick Douglass Memorial Hospital in Philadelphia. The creation of the Freedmen's Hospital in Washington and the work of early African American medical workers in Washington helped lead to a national infrastructure of African American academic medicine. *Courtesy of the National Library of Medicine.*

First published 2014

Manufactured in the United States

ISBN 978.1.62619.655.1

Library of Congress Control Number: 2014951893

To Colonel Robert Gould Shaw and the brave men of the Fifty-fourth Massachusetts who started me on this path, to Dr. Alexander Thomas Augusta for helping me complete this journey and to all the men and women who have served their country so valiantly.

CONTENTS

FOREWORD

Professor Heather Butts's interest in this topic was piqued as she gained increasing knowledge about the problematic healthcare issues relative to Americans of African ancestry that date back to slavery. Further consideration for a book project drew perpetual concerns from those who questioned the amount of effort required. Butts did not deny her uncertainties but still was driven by the need to address a basic issue of human well-being and survival. Illuminating the historical role of African American healthcare providers tells the edifying story of initiative, responsibility, determination and empowerment. However daunting, pursuing the challenge became an unshakable commitment, and the predecessor of this work was begun several years back.

Professor Butts's academic preparation, including completing her undergraduate/graduate studies at Princeton, St. John's Law School, Harvard School of Public Health and Columbia University School of Education/Psychology, established a solid foundation for her research pursuits. Combined with various work experiences, the creation of for-profit and nonprofit organizations and engaging in hours of research on the project made her well prepared for the task she undertook as the author of this work. It clearly reflects legal, physical, psychological, public health and educational focuses that offer an inspiring multidisciplinarian orientation to her material.

Her study is complex as she examines the Washington, D.C.–based African Americans who participated in combat as well as those who provided healthcare during the Civil War. Butts points out the fact that thousands of African Americans died during the Civil War. Pneumonia, dysentery, typhoid fever and malaria accounted for the majority of medical deaths.

Both white soldiers and civilians resisted any participation by African Americans in the war effort. On August 8, 1862, General Sherman ordered that African American soldiers be employed as cooks, laborers and nurses, not as combat soldiers.

It is my contention that current healthcare issues challenging the African American community are rooted in the dehumanizing physical, psychological and emotional treatment of African Americans. This occurred before, during and after the Civil War. I have concerns about the health conditions of African Americans who are confronting yet another survival issue.

The African American family is a significant social institution that introduces organization and structure to its members. At this point in American history, we can document a past besieged by atrocious practices that served to reduce the quality of life for many African American families. There are dire consequences related to these inadequacies, most notably an insufficient or total lack of healthcare.

Butts's study examines the interplay between slaves and others of African ancestry and their roles in the context of the Civil War. The determination and contributions of African American soldiers, doctors and healthcare providers is documented. Selecting Washington, D.C., as a focal point to explore reflects the significance of its geographic location and its role as the seat of government for the nation. It provides, too, an awareness of healthcare of African American family life over the past three centuries.

As an African American physician, I am very proud of and thankful for the myriad exemplary early contributions made by African American healthcare providers as addressed in this work. Butts deserves scores of accolades for her enlightenment regarding this momentous period in American history.

Hugh F. Butts, MD

PREFACE

In 1863, Dr. Alexander T. Augusta wrote a detailed letter to Abraham Lincoln requesting an appointment as a surgeon in the Union army: "I beg leave to apply to you for an appointment as surgeon to some of the coloured regiments, or as physician to some of the depots of freedom." Having left the United States in the 1850s to gain admittance to medical school, Augusta was a successful businessman and physician in Toronto, and he and his wife lived the life of a professional African American family in Canada. Augusta had no reason to upend his tranquil, successful life and volunteer his medical services to Lincoln and the Union army. Except, he did have a reason, several in fact—duty, honor and valor. Augusta, as will become evident in this book, was a man of honor. He was a man of valor who believed he had a duty to his country to be a part of this important effort.

While there has been a fair amount of scholarship in recent years around the role that African Americans played in the war from a fighting perspective, the role that they played as healthcare workers has received limited review. Additionally, their healthcare picture and the care they received during the war has also lacked scholarly analysis. Specifically, the role that Washington, D.C., had is deserving of examination. This book hopes to add to this discourse and, to a certain extent, give voice to those who cared for African Americans during the war and those African Americans who cared for the sick and the wounded.

ACKNOWLEDGEMENTS

I first became interested in writing about this area of history as a student at Harvard University's School of Public Health in 1997–98. I was doing research on Civil War medicine and happened on an entry in a book about Dr. Alexander Augusta, an African American Civil War surgeon. My interest grew, and in 2005, I authored an article about Augusta for the *Journal of the National Medical Association*. Almost ten years later, I am proud to know that the story of Dr. Augusta, as well as so many other courageous men and women, will be told in this publication.

I am extremely grateful to my loving family who fully supported my efforts from the inception of this book until its conclusion. My mother, Clementine R. Butts, LCSW, was facilitator and problem solver to get the work done, and my father, Hugh F. Butts, MD, provided insightful consultation. My sisters—Sydney C. Butts, MD, FACS, never allowed me to compromise on my goal to achieve excellence, and Samantha F. Butts, MD, MSCE, established positive alternatives as a means of helping to maintain a balance in my life. My entire family has always modeled the kind of courage and valor that I hope I have conveyed through my writing this book.

To my dear friends and proofreaders—a deep appreciation to Professor Margaret Turano for her constructive guidance and enduring support and for reading more versions of this book than any one person should be required to read; Anthony Antonucci, who gave feedback, rigorously questioned aspects of the text and encouraged me to progress and finish the text; renowned author Harriet Washington, who was convinced that this project would see the light of day and, thus, urged me to stay the course; and Cliff E. Barnes, Esq., my astute Washingtonian mentor who advised about the timeliness of the book. Lu Willard and Stanley Hoffman began creating public interest in the book well ahead of its arrival. David A. Brockway maintained a listening ear, always ready to be an objective sounding board. Robert J. Ruben, MD, has greatly enhanced the quality of my life from early childhood. Cheryl Hill shared some interesting early history about members of her Washington family in the healthcare field. Alan Miller, MD, has been a wonderful mentor whose commitment to public health work inspired me to pursue that academic path. I thank Marita G. Monroe for her efforts in promoting this important work. To my board and staff family at the Northside Center for Child Development—you inspire me daily with your commitment to helping others. I also thank Judith Nigro, Diana Dell, Carol Dingle, so many devoted extended family members, friends and my loyal Kew Forest family.

Thank you to those who supported this project even before it was the project it has turned into today—Dr. Ida E. Jones of Howard University, who provided me with a pivotal piece of research years ago, which led to my first article on this subject a decade ago; Dr. Frank Smith of the African American Civil War Memorial and Museum, who supported my article on Dr. Augusta and encouraged me to continue with my research; and my professors, students and mentors at Princeton University, Harvard University, Saint John's Law School and Columbia University, all of whom supported my work in different ways.

Of course, so many thanks go to my amazing editor Banks Smither. His patience and support were invaluable. He has been a consummate professional and positive presence during this endeavor. My appreciation also goes to Katie Stitely, the project editor at The History Press whose insightful work on this project enhanced the final product immeasurably. Thank you to everyone at The History Press for their talent, patience and support.

I hope you enjoy this publication that I believe has importance for all of us as a nation. I hope that this inspires those who read it to delve even more deeply into this important piece of our country's history.

1

African American Healthcare Providers and Patients in D.C. Prior to the Civil War

While the majority of African American healthcare providers' D.C. stories began during the war, some of them had contact with the city before the conflict. This chapter examines those providers as well as the overall state of African American healthcare before the war, particularly in D.C.

Washington, D.C., was an interesting town prior to the Civil War. In 1830, over half of the African Americans in Washington, D.C., were free. By 1850, free African Americans outnumbered enslaved African Americans by two to one. D.C. had "black codes" regulating the conduct and opportunities that were available to free African Americans.

The first black codes were instituted in 1808 and involved curfews that resulted in fines of five dollars. Unpaid fines resulted in individuals being whipped. Black codes increased in harshness in 1812 when fines increased to twenty dollars and unpaid fines were punished with six months' jail time. African Americans in D.C. were subject to 10:00 p.m. curfews and morality laws, such as being unable to gamble, play cards or curse in public. African Americans in D.C. had very few political rights, could not testify against whites in court and had to carry documents confirming their status as free individuals at all times.[1] In 1821, additional codes were imposed on free African Americans. Black codes hindered but did not prevent a number of African Americans from prospering as restaurant owners and merchants. Others worked at a variety of trades and service occupations, including bricklayers, painters, shoemakers, nurses and physicians.[2]

The D.C. Compensation Act of April 16, 1862, ended slavery in D.C. and freed over 3,100 enslaved individuals. The act also reimbursed slave owners and offered newly freed slaves money to emigrate to other countries.[3] In 1800, 25 percent of D.C.'s population was African American, and the vast majority of them were enslaved. Slaves also earned freedom in D.C. through the death of slaves' owners who granted freedom in their wills.[4] These numbers grew with time, and as African Americans labored on projects like building the White House and Capitol, they were able to buy their freedom and live in D.C. as free men and women. Thousands of slaves fled to D.C., and consequently, the Contraband Camp in D.C. was established. Historian Jill Newmark described the hospital:

> *On a parcel of swampy land in northwest Washington, D.C. bounded by 12th, 13th, R and S streets, NW, a tented camp and hospital once stood that served thousands of escaped slaves and black soldiers during the Civil War. Known as Contraband Camp, it contained one of the few hospitals that treated blacks in Washington, D.C. during the war and whose staff including nurses and surgeons, were largely African American.*[5]

According to Elizabeth Keckley, dressmaker and confidante to first lady Mary Todd Lincoln:

> *They came with a great hope in their hearts, and with all their worldly goods on their backs...the north is not warm and impulsive. The bright joyous dreams of freedom to the slave—faded—were sadly altered in the presence of that stern, practical mother, reality. Poor dusky children of slavery, men and women, of my own race—the transition from slavery to freedom was too sudden for you.*[6]

Among the issues faced by free African Americans were 10:00 p.m. curfews and morality laws seeking to legislate their behavior. With the influx of so many African American "contrabands" to Washington, D.C., shelters were constructed, first on Capitol Hill, then the U Street Corridor and eventually in Arlington County. Services such as education and healthcare began and recruitment of service members took place.[7]

It was in the face of this that healthcare issues, with respect to African Americans, surfaced. Many of these issues had their inception in slavery and in the transition for African Americans from a system of servitude to a status of freedom. This transition was more difficult for some than others and particularly difficult in a city such as Washington, D.C.

HEALTHCARE OF AFRICAN AMERICANS IN D.C.

The toll that slavery took on both the slaves that endured the system and those who propagated it is incalculable. Information on the health of African Americans before the war is available by looking at the health of African Americans who enlisted in the war. It is critical to understand the health status of African Americans prior to the war in order to understand their health outcomes during the war.

According to English legal academic and author Edward Strutt Abdy, who visted Washington in the 1830s:

> *One day I went to see the slave pen—a wretched hovel "right again" the Capitol, from which it is distant about half a mile, with no house intervening...At a small window above, which was unglazed and exposed alike to heat of summer and the cold of winter, so trying to the constitution, two or three sable faces appeared, looking out wistfully to while away the time and catch a refreshing breeze; the weather being extremely hot.*[8]

The hardships that African Americans had to endure while living in slavery through the 1850s took a physical and psychological toll on their health. Additionally, as African American slaves in Washington, D.C., became older and sicker, their utility lessened, and they were often reduced to begging for money to earn their keep. The usefulness of a slave was in his or her ability to be productive, and that meant being as healthy as possible, under the circumstances.

Factors such as a poor living standard, the amount and level of work and the lack of access to healthcare led to high mortality rates for slaves.[9] According to the 1850 census, the average age of death for African Americans was 21.4 years as opposed to 25.5 years for whites. In 1860, 3.5 percent of slaves and 4.4 percent of whites were over the age of sixty.[10]

All experiences slaves had with a doctor or nurse were under the control of their owner. Physicians often had a contract with the slave owner to care for all the slaves on a plantation. The most obvious difference between healthcare for whites and slaves was that slaves did not have control over their own bodies. Moreover, the slave "body" was the economic engine that kept the southern economy in place. It was up to the slave owner to decide, in conjunction with the doctor, the medical course of treatment for that slave. Slaves had to report all illnesses to their owners. This, in turn, created an interesting paradox where slaves who became ill would often try to self-medicate with herbs or roots. If the illness persisted, they were forced to tell their owner of the sickness and that they had self-medicated. This would often be an indication to the owner that the slave had little interest in his or her own health or the health of his or her children. Exacerbating the healthcare problems for many slaves was that they lived in close quarters and were exposed to parasites, bacteria, human waste and garbage.

It is important to chronicle the healthcare of slaves during slavery because it is within this context that many intergenerational disease processes were inherited from African Americans in the 1800s, both for free African Americans and slaves. Under this umbrella of healthcare of slaves, we can transition to examine healthcare for African Americans during the Civil War.

It does appear that there was a cohort of African Americans, namely older slaves, that had, if not better, at least comparable health outcomes to their white counterparts. There are several reasons for this.[11] First, older slaves were those who had been able to avoid deadly childhood and midlife illnesses and life-threatening accidents. They might have developed a healthcare-coping mechanism that allowed them to successfully reach old age. If a slave reached a mature age, it was financially wise to keep the slave healthy and alive, either for work or sale.[12] Slaves also developed mechanisms of keeping older slaves healthy.

The psychological impact of slavery cannot be denied. The lack of mental health services for African Americans in the 1800s has led to a "legacy of neglect" for African Americans' mental health issues today.[13] This, coupled with the psychological trauma that African Americans went through during slavery, led to generational tension with mental health and treatment. During the 1800s, the main mental health diagnoses for all individuals were melancholy, mania, dementia and idiocy. For slaves however, *drapetomania* and *dysaethesia aethiopicia* were the diagnoses of choice.

Drapetomia, characterized by being sulky and dissatisfied, often "resulted" in slave escape and runaway situations. Many of these diagnoses were premised on the notion that slaves were unjustifiably dissatisfied with their place in life and irrationally decided to run away from a perfectly good slave master and home where they were taken care of.[14]

Dysaethesia aethiopicia was defined as mischief, poor work habits or destruction of property. According to Tony Lowe, while environmental factors were attributed to mental health issues of whites in the 1800s, social inferiority and biological defects were the etiology many attributed to African Americans' mental health issues. Some doctors even suggested that slavery helped to ameliorate such inherent mental health issues.[15] The stigma attached to slaves, coupled with a need to justify the institution, led to such notions.

The slave narrative entitled *The Life of Gustavus Vassa* tells the story of how slave masters neglected and cruelly treated slaves.

> *One Mr. D—— told me he had sold 41,000 negroes and he once cut off a negro-man's leg for running away. I asked him if the man had died in the operation, how he, as a Christian, could answer, for the horrid act before God...He...said that his scheme had the desired effect—it cured that man and some others of running away.*[16]

The narrative goes on to describe the health of slaves, stating:

> *Another negro-man was half hanged, and then burnt, for attempting to poison a cruel overseer. Thus by repeated cruelties, are the wretched first urged to despair, and then murdered, because they still retain so much of human nature about them as to wish to put an end to their misery, and to retaliate on their tyrants! Their overseers are, indeed, for the most part, persons of the worst character of any denomination of men in the West Indies. Unfortunately, many humane gentlemen, but not residing on their estates, are obliged to leave the management of them in the hands of these human butchers, who cut and mangle the slaves in a shocking manner, on the most trivial occasions, and altogether treat them, in every respect, like brutes. They pay no regard to the situation of pregnant women, nor the least attention to the lodging of the field negroes. Their huts, which ought to be well covered, and the place dry where they take their short repose, are often open sheds, guilt in damp places; so that, when the poor creatures return tired from the toils of the field, they contract many disorders, from being exposed to the damp*

> *air in this uncomfortable state, while they are heated, and their pores are open. The neglect certainly conspires with many others to cause a decrease in the births as well as in the lives of the grown negroes.*[17]

From a public health perspective, there is a question about the health of African Americans as they entered the war. How does one quantify the level of health for this population? One way to do this would be childhood health. Another way would be by using height indicators. In *A Peculiar Population: The Nutrition, Health, and Mortality of American Slaves from Childhood to Maturity*, Richard H. Steckel does an exhaustive review of the height and mortality data of slaves.[18]

In 1807, Congress passed legislation requiring ship captains to describe each slave based on name, age, sex, color and height.[19] Because the need for good nutrition increases dramatically during adolescence, it is instructive to identify the average age of growth spurt in the slave population. It appears that the peak of the adolescent growth spurt for female slaves was 13.27 years and for male slaves 14.75 years, approximately 1–1.15 years behind that of averages for individuals, regardless of race, during that time period.[20] It is clear that young slave children were well below the expected height levels. But there is an interesting phenomenon with slaves as they matured—they essentially made up for their height disparities in their teenage years and into adulthood.[21]

Slaves caught up with respect to growth. By age sixteen and a half, for example, American male slaves were taller than factory workers and laboring classes in England, factory workers in Russia and German peasants.[22]

It is provoking to think about the seeming incongruity between childhood height rates and adolescent growth spurts among slaves. Why were slave children so small? Much of this can be traced to birth rates and birth weights. Slave newborns, on average, weighed five and one-half pounds. Once born, these infants had a poor diet after breast-feeding, which led to high infant mortality and sickness rates. If a baby made it through infancy, then he or she had to deal with a poor diet as a child. Slave masters focused on working slaves and their diets, not the children's. Slave owners did a cost-benefit analysis: If slave children made it into late childhood and early adolescence, the return on investment at that point was worth the money to the slave masters.[23]

The focus on the laborer in the slave system influenced slaves themselves. If the thought was that the adult laborer was the modern equivalent of the "bread winner," then the entire family was invested in the health and strength of that family member, even to the detriment of younger family members. Slaves made up their height differential when they joined the labor force. This corresponds with an improved diet and the slave owner's including meat in the slave's diet once he or she became a laborer.[24]

Unlike other societies where individuals continued to be poorly nourished through adulthood, when slaves entered the workforce, they were deemed to be a cost-benefit to their masters and, thus, deserving of a better diet, or at least a diet that included meat. This seems to have been an important factor in spurring growth among slave adolescents.

Below is a quote from Walt Whitman which manifests his views on slavery:

> *I say where* LIBERTY DRAWS NOT THE BLOOD OUT OF SLAVERY, THERE SLAVERY DRAWS THE BLOOD OUT OF LIBERTY. *After all, I may have been trained a bit, just a little bit with the New York feeling with regard to anti-slavery. The horror of slavery always had a strong hold on me. Slavery and the tremendous spreading of hands to protect it and the stern opposition to it which shall never cease, or the speaking of tongues and the moving of lips ceases. I observe the slights and degradations cast by arrogant persons upon laborers, the poor and upon African Americans, and the like. Or I guess the grass itself is a child…a uniform hieroglyphic…growing among black folks as among white…large fine headed nobly formed superbly destined, on equal terms with me! Everyone who speaks his word for slavery is himself the worst slave—the spirit of freeman is not light enough to show him that all the fatness of earth were bitter to a bondaged neck—when a feast I eat corn and roast potatoes for my dinner through my own voluntary choice, it is very well and I am much content, but if some arrogant head of the table prevent me by force from touching anything but corn and potatoes then is my anger aroused. I was a decided and outspoken anti-slavery believer myself then and always but steered from the extremist, the red hot fellows of these times.*[25]

Whitman's attitude on slavery was further expressed in a dispatch to the *Brooklyn Daily Eagle*, dated March 18, 1856:

> *Public attention within the last few days has been naturally turned to the slave trade—that most abominable of all man's schemes for making money without regard to the character of the means used for the purpose.*

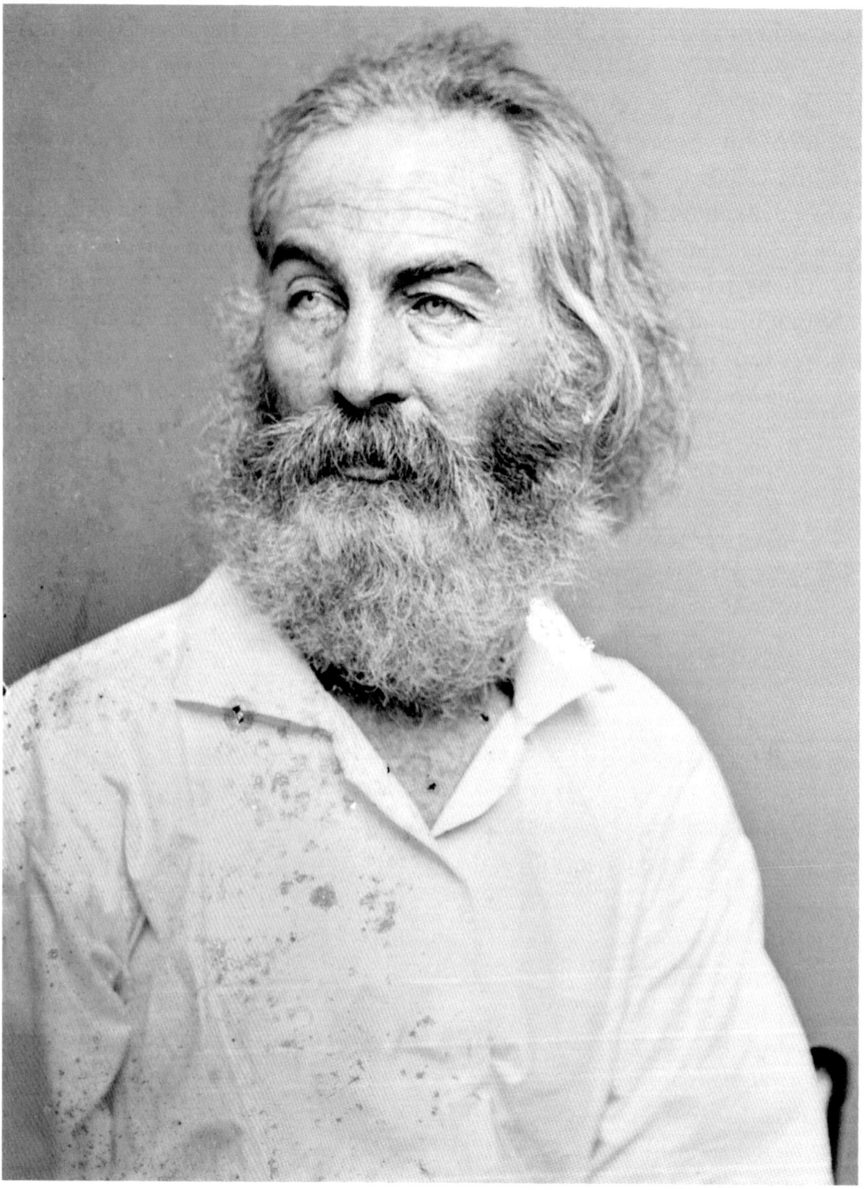

Walt Whitman, author and Washington, D.C. Civil War nurse. *Courtesy of the Library of Congress, Washington, D.C.*

Four vessels have, in about as many days, been brought to the American territory for being engaged in this monstrous business! It is a disgrace and a blot on the character of our Republic and on our biased humanity! Though we hear less nowadays of this trade—of the atrocious slave hunt—of the crowding of a mass of compact human flesh into little more than its own equal in space—we are not to suppose that such horrors have ceased to exist. The great nations—our own first of all—have passed stringent laws against the slave traffic. But Brazil encourages it still. And many citizens of Europe and America pursue it notwithstanding its illegality. Still the African American is torn from his simple hut—from his children, his brethren, his parents and friends to be carried far away and made the bondsman of a stranger. Still the black hearted traitors who ply this work go forth with their armed bands and swoop down on the defenseless villages and bring their loads of human trophy, chained and gagged, and sell them as so much merchandise! The slave-ship! How few of our readers know the beginning of the horrors involved in that term! Imagine a vessel of the fourth or fifth class, built more for speed than space, and therefore with narrow accommodations even for a few passengers; a space between decks divided into two compartments, three feet, three inches from floor to ceiling—one of these compartments sixteen feet by eight, the other forty by twenty-one- the first holding two hundred and twenty-six children and youth of both sexes, the second, three hundred and thirty-six men and women and all this is a latitude where the thermometer is at eight degrees in the shade. Are you sick of the description? O, this is not all by a good sight. Imagine neither food nor water given these hapless prisoners except a little of the latter, at long intervals, which they spill in their mad eagerness to get it; many of the women advanced in pregnancy—the motion of the seas sickening those who have never before felt it—dozens of the poor wretches dying, and others already dead (and they are most to be envied!)—the very air so thick that the lungs cannot perform their office—and all this for filthy lucre! Pah! We are almost a misanthrope to our kind when we think they will do such things! Of the nine hundred Negroes (there were doubtless more) originally on board the Pons, *not six hundred and fifty remained when she arrived back and landed her inmates at Monrovia! It is enough to make the heart pause its pulsation to read the scene presented at the liberation of these sons of misery.—Most of them were boys, of from twelve to twenty years. What woe must have spread through many an African American mother's heart from this wicked business! It is not ours to find an excuse for slaving in the benighted condition whose horrors we have been describing—did not facts prove the contrary. The "middle passage" is yet going on with all its deadly crime and cruelty. The slave trade yet exists. Why? The laws are sharp enough, too sharp. But who ever heard of their being put in force, further than to confiscate the vessel, and perhaps imprison the crews a few days? But the laws should pry out every man who helps the slave trade—not merely the sailor on the sea, but the cowardly rich villain and speculator on the land—and punish him. It cannot be effectually stopped until that is done—and Brazil forced by the black muzzles of American and European men-of-war cannot to stop her part of the business too. To the American young men, mechanics, farmers, etc. How much longer do you intend to submit to the espionage and terrorism of the three hundred and fifty thousand owners of slaves? Are you too their slaves and their most obedient slaves? Shall no one among you dare open his mouth to say he is opposed to slavery, as a man should be on account of the whites, and want it abolished for their sake? Is not a writer, speaker, teacher to be left alive but those who lick the spit that drops from the mouths of the three hundred fifty thousand masters? Is there hardly one free, courageous soul left in fifteen large and populous states? Do the ranks of the owners of slaves themselves contain no men desperate and tired of that services and sweat of the mind, worse than any of that service in sugar fields or cornfields.*[26]

AFRICAN AMERICAN HEALTHCARE PROVIDERS TRAINING AND WORKING IN D.C.

As author Todd Savitt points out, after the Civil War and into the early twentieth century, the majority of African American physicians graduated from medical schools founded by African Americans. Whereas pre–Civil War, African Americans wishing to pursue medicine often had to resort to studying in Canada, post–Civil War, more schools accepted African Americans.[27] An example of the trajectory of African Americans and their training prior to the war can be seen in Dr. Alexander Augusta.

Dr. Alexander Augusta secretly learned to read, with the help of Bishop Daniel Payne and, by the 1840s, had moved to Baltimore, Maryland, to begin studying medicine with private tutors while he worked as a barber.[28] According to Dr. Montague Cobb, who wrote one of the definitive articles on Dr. Augusta, "He obtained his early education by stealth from [Episcopalian] Bishop Payne, as it was then against the law to teach colored persons."[29]

Augusta worked with Dr. William Gibson of the University of Pennsylvania. In much the same way that apprentice relationships worked in the 1800s, Augusta was able to learn from Gibson and gain knowledge about the craft that he hoped one day to call his profession—namely, medicine. With the encouragement of Gibson, he attempted to gain admittance to the University of Pennsylvania's Medical School; however, in what would be an ongoing theme in Augusta's life, he was denied admittance and had to look elsewhere to pursue his education. The first African American to gain admittance to the University of Pennsylvania's Medical School would be Nathan Francis Mossell.[30] Mossell wrote his autobiography at the age of ninety. In his own words, he states that:

> *In the fall of 1879* [I] *made formal application for admission to the opening session of the School of Medicine. I was promptly informed...that the department had never admitted a colored student...At a subsequent date...I was called and was informed that the faculty voted in my favor.*[31]

Dr. Mossell would go on to be the founder of Frederick Douglass Memorial Hospital, a place in the mode of hospitals such as Freedmen's Hospital in D.C., and, in Mossell's own words, "a place where young colored women could train for nursing; I was particular to explode the taboo against women physicians in hospital management. Women physicians were associated with Douglass Hospital from its inception."[32]

It was important for doctors in the mid- to late 1800s to obtain additional training in the form of apprenticeships, as this was one way to become an allopathic physician. For African American physicians, this was an inordinately difficult task to achieve in the United States. Augusta continued to study with Gibson, but he knew that his true passion was to continue his training in an academic setting.

The commencement of the Civil War had a profound effect on Augusta.[33] From his early days in the Baltimore/D.C. area, he was a staunch supporter of the rights of African Americans. Augusta's desire to pursue his dream of going to medical school did not dampen his deep-seated need to be a champion for human rights generally and African Americans' rights specifically. Augusta was an avid supporter of antislavery

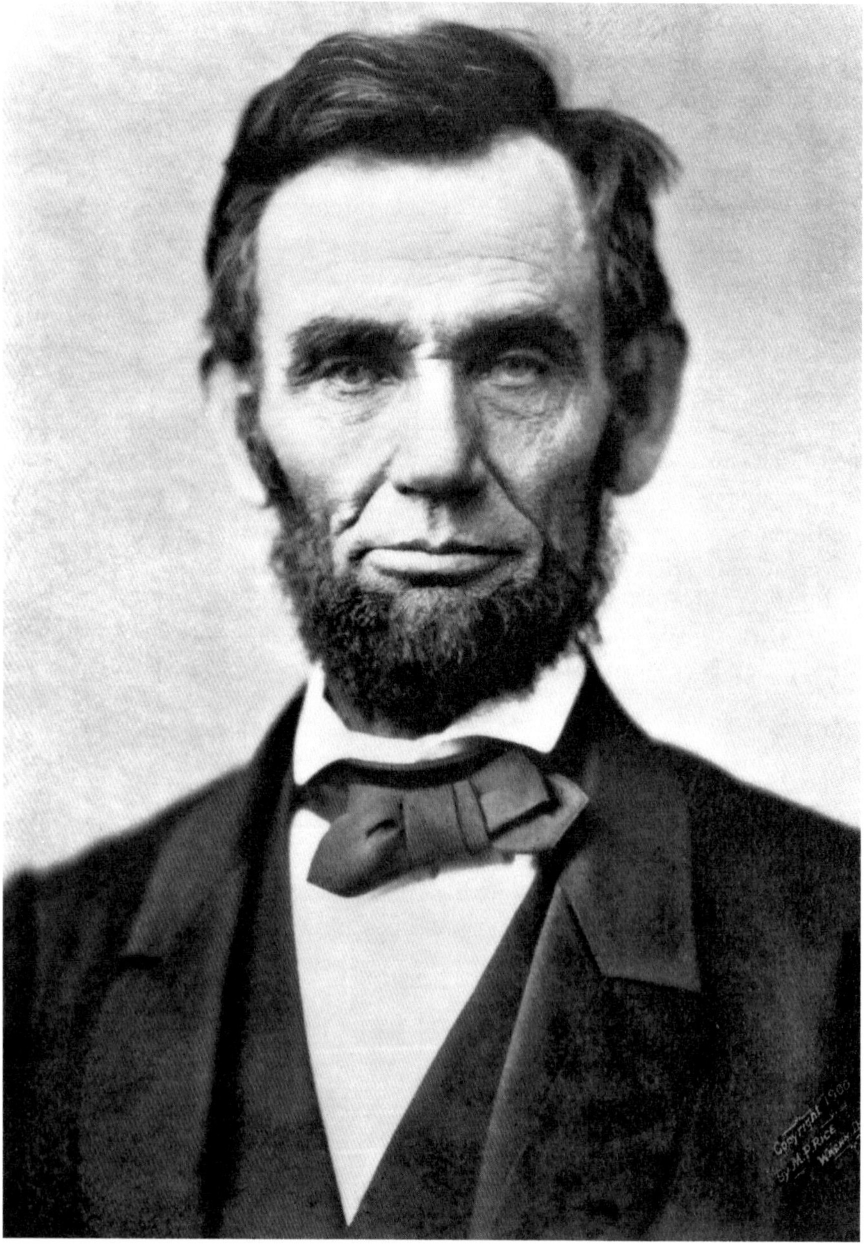

President Abraham Lincoln. *Courtesy of the Library of Congress, Washington, D.C.*

Opposite: The Capitol under construction prior to the Civil War. *Courtesy of the United States National Archives and Records Administration.*

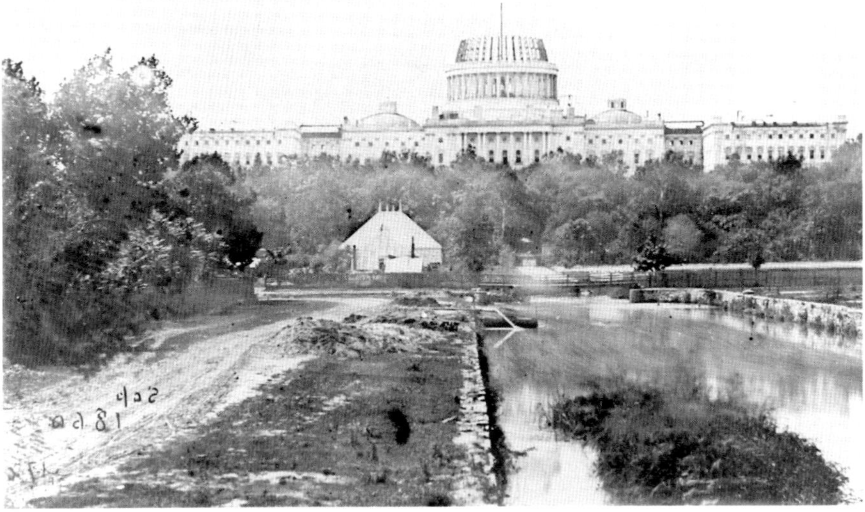

causes while in Canada, and it was his devotion to freedom for fellow African Americans that compelled him to return to Washington, D.C., at the beginning of the Civil War and participate in the war efforts in whatever way possible. Augusta wrote letters to Abraham Lincoln and Edwin Stanton requesting an appointment as a surgeon or physician for one of the African American regiments formed by the Union army: "I beg leave to apply to you for an appointment as surgeon to some of the coloured regiments, or as physician to some of the depots of 'freedmen.' I was compelled to leave my native country, and come to this on account of prejudices against colour, for the purpose of obtaining a knowledge of my profession; and having accomplished that object, at one of the principle educational institutions of this province, I am now prepared to practice it, and would like to be a position where I can be of use to my race."[34]

Washington, D.C., was not only an unusual city when the Civil War began but also a city in flux. According to author Glenna Schroeder-Lein, the Capitol building had no dome and the wings for the Senate and House of Representatives were not complete.[35] According to the Census Bureau, in 1850, the overall population was 51,687, with 37,941 of those individuals being white and 13,746 of those individuals being African American. Of those individuals, 10,059 were free and 3,687 were enslaved. By 1860, those numbers were 75,080 overall, with 60,763 white and 13,746 African American. The enslaved population in 1860 for D.C. was 3,185, and the free population was

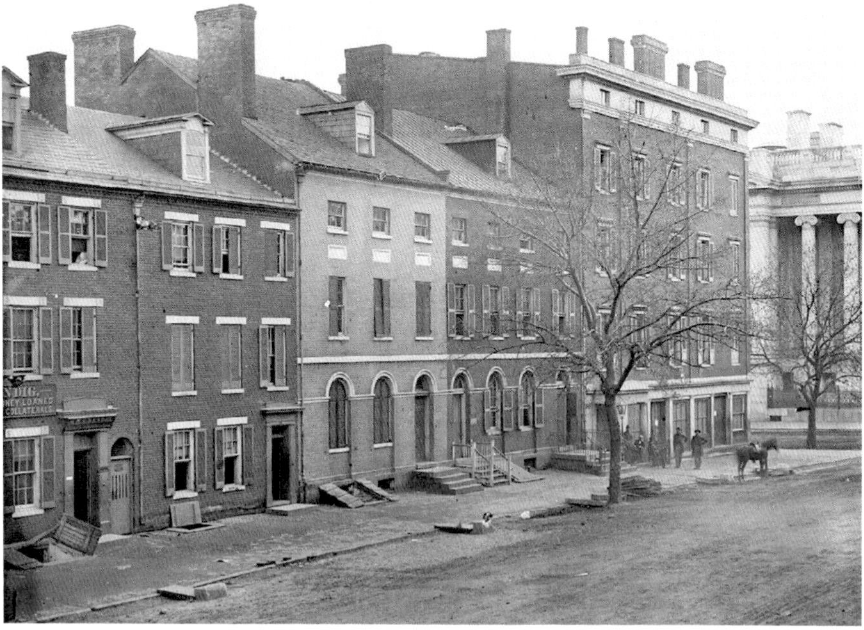

Fifteenth and F Streets in Washington, D.C., near the streetcar incident Dr. Augusta was in. *Courtesy of the Library of Congress, Washington, D.C.*

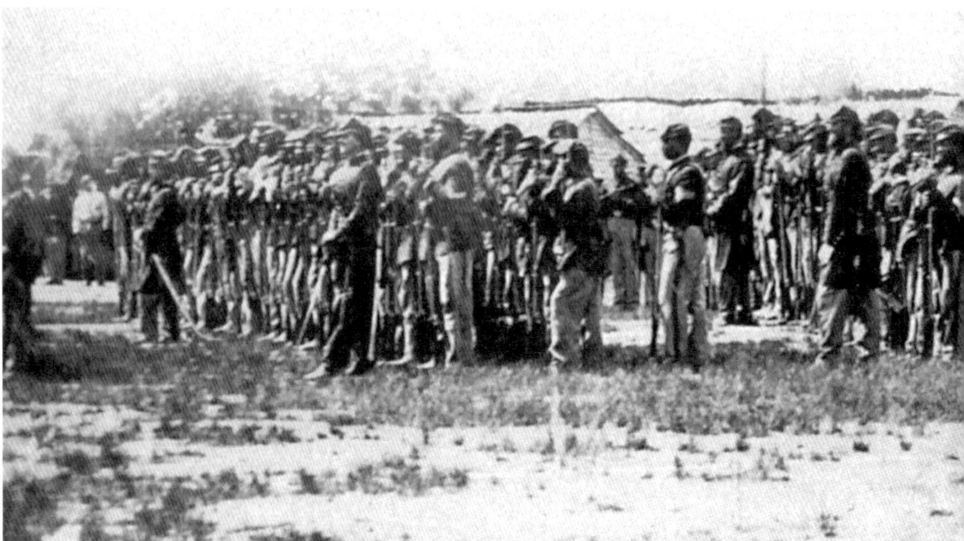

African American soldiers of the First Regiment of the United States Colored Infantry training in Washington, D.C. *Courtesy of the University of North Florida.*

11,131.[36] It was under these circumstances that African American surgeons came to practice in Washington, D.C., during the war. It is important to note that because the vast majority of African Americans wishing to serve as physicians during the war had to find alternative methods of obtaining their medical training (including leaving the country), very few physicians who served during the war have professional ties to D.C. prior to the war.

On April 14, 1863, Augusta was appointed surgeon of the United States Colored Troops (USCT). After Augusta received his commission, he was sent to Camp Barker in Washington, D.C. For many officers in the Union army, although they believed in spirit that there should be equality for all, they had few dealings with African Americans. Several lower-ranking officers were perplexed as to how to deal with a higher-ranking African American officer.[37]

Henry Turner was born in Newberry, South Carolina, a free man. His grandmother taught him to read and write, and he got a job cleaning at a law office where he gained the notice of the lawyers in the firm who supported his education. In 1853, Turner was licensed to preach, and he ended up ministering in both white and African American churches. In 1858, Turner joined the African Methodist Episcopal Church (AME). The senior AME bishop, Daniel Payne, arranged for Turner to go to Baltimore to further

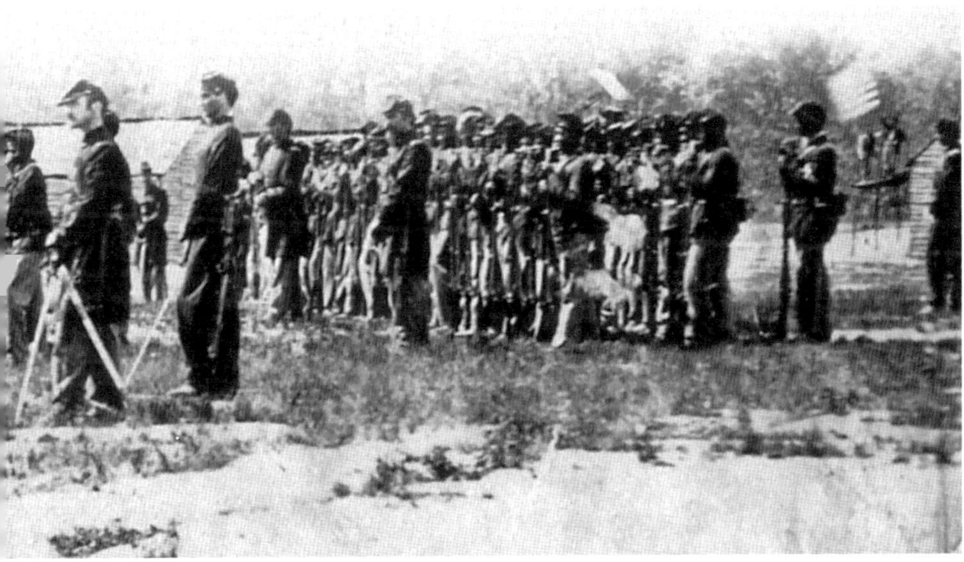

his studies. When the Civil War broke out, Turner was in Baltimore and began to support African Americans who wanted to fight in the war. Turner became a recruiter of soldiers in D.C. in the early 1860s and received a commission as chaplain of the First United States Colored Troops.[38] This regiment was organized in the spring and summer of 1863 in Washington, D.C., and trained at Analostan Island.[39]

According to author Edwin Redkey:

> *In Washington, Turner recruited vigorously for the local unit, urging both free born and "contrabands" to enlist in the 1st USCT. While the men trained, he came regularly to preach for them, reminding them that the destiny of their race depended on their loyalty and courage. On occasion the regiment marched in body to Israel AME Church to hear one of his patriotic sermons. In July 1863 the regiment, having filled its quota of a thousand men, prepared to leave for the war zone. By this time an African American clergyman had already been commissioned in the 55th Massachusetts Volunteer Infantry Regiment. Turner having urged black men to risk their lives to free the slaves, began campaigning to get himself appointed chaplain of the Washington regiment. In November, at the age of thirty, he finally received his commission, becoming the only black officer in the 1st USCT.*[40]

2

Unique Healthcare Issues of African American Soldiers and Prisoners of War

For the most part, operations and surgical procedures during the Civil War were not elective.[41] The average Union soldier wounded in a battle was usually shot in the arm or leg by a soft lead bullet fired from a musket. Chances were high that he would not survive.[42] Many Union doctors were not prepared for surgery in war conditions and learned how to treat gunshot wounds and perform amputations on the job.[43]

Thousands of African American soldiers died in the Civil War, with the vast majority of African American service members dying from illness.[44] Pneumonia, dysentery, typhoid fever and malaria took the heaviest tolls on the African American ranks. Within specific commands, the number of deaths was quite stark. An African American heavy artillery regiment lost over eight hundred men, and one infantry regiment, in service less than one year, had 524 deaths, which was nearly 50 percent of the regiment.[45] According to author John MacDonald:

> *Sick and wounded from the battlefields poured into Washington throughout the war. The arrival* [at the] *Sixth Street dock in May 1862 of the steamer* Louisiana *with 213 sick soldiers from the Peninsular Campaign brought the number of convalescents sent to Washington from the front to about 1,600. Some were dying of consumption. In a few instances, the nearest relatives were on hand to greet them. The Washington Star noted that only the sick had been sent to Washington's hospitals; the wounded had been sent by boat to other Northern cities. Washington had 21 hospitals to treat wounded*

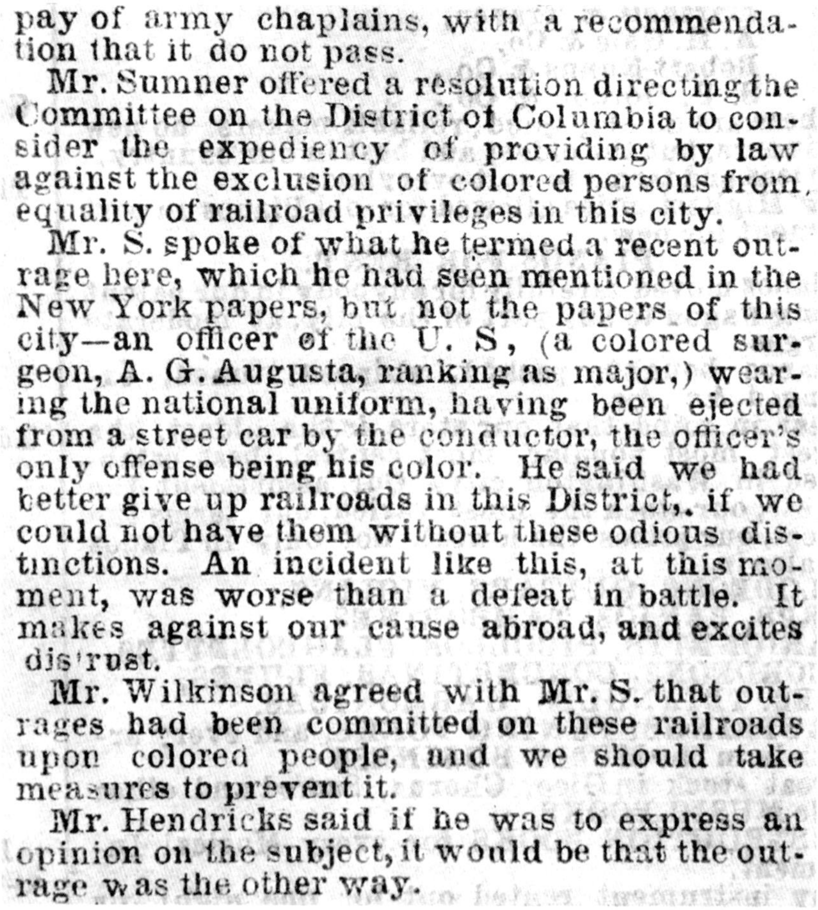

pay of army chaplains, with a recommendation that it do not pass.

Mr. Sumner offered a resolution directing the Committee on the District of Columbia to consider the expediency of providing by law against the exclusion of colored persons from equality of railroad privileges in this city.

Mr. S. spoke of what he termed a recent outrage here, which he had seen mentioned in the New York papers, but not the papers of this city—an officer of the U. S, (a colored surgeon, A. G. Augusta, ranking as major,) wearing the national uniform, having been ejected from a street car by the conductor, the officer's only offense being his color. He said we had better give up railroads in this District, if we could not have them without these odious distinctions. An incident like this, at this moment, was worse than a defeat in battle. It makes against our cause abroad, and excites distrust.

Mr. Wilkinson agreed with Mr. S. that outrages had been committed on these railroads upon colored people, and we should take measures to prevent it.

Mr. Hendricks said if he was to express an opinion on the subject, it would be that the outrage was the other way.

A description of Dr. Alexander Augusta's commission in the Union army. *Courtesy of the District of Columbia Public Library.*

soldiers, some of them located in the Patent Office; churches and public halls. Wounded…came by train and boat from savage battles such as Fredericksburg and Chancellorsville in Virginia. The walking wounded, bandaged, disheveled and blackened with gunpowder smoke, often had to fend for themselves until they reached a hospital…On occasion, doctors were brought into the city from the nearby States of Pennsylvania, Maryland and Delaware in order to tend the sick and wounded. Soldiers discharged from the hospitals were sent to Camp Convalescent in Alexandria, where deplorable conditions existed.[46]

An important factor regarding the healthcare of African Americans was the quality of physicians who served in their regiments. It was difficult to find surgeons willing to serve with African American regiments. Further, the military was reluctant to have African Americans serve as doctors in these regiments. According to Major General Banks, "In the organization of the colored regiments there was a serious want of Surgeons. Competent men declined to enter the service. It was impossible to get good officers to accept such commissions." According to the general, "In very many cases, Hospital Stewards of low order of qualification were appointed to the office of assistant surgeon and Surgeon. Well-grounded objections were made from every quarter against the inhumanity of subjecting the colored soldiers to medical treatment and surgical operations by such men. It...could not be disregarded without bringing discredit upon the Army and the Government."[47]

African American soldiers were not alone in being subject to the care of less-than-competent surgeons or individuals who were not surgeons at all. White soldiers could fully expect the same treatment in a difficult battle with few resources. It was left to the army to discover creative ways to find qualified medical care for the African American soldiers. Physician J.V.C. Smith was asked to go to the medical schools through the country to scout out possible medical providers for the African American regiments, and he did so with a certain degree of success.[48] Smith, a prominent doctor, toured particularly throughout New England in search of possible surgeons for the war effort.[49]

According to a white physician in the United States Colored Infantry (USCI), "Very few surgeons will do precisely the same for African Americans as they would for whites."[50] African American patients often complained of being treated very callously.

In another case, a surgeon in the Fifth USCI failed to attend to the needs of an African American soldier whose foot had been partially severed by a shell because he was conducting sick call. Sick call refers to the daily lineup of soldiers who require medical attention. Medical personnel are required to record the treatment they provide the soldiers and fill out a record of treatment for each patient they care for. The doctor defended himself by stating that "a man with a part of his foot cut off by a piece of shell was not suffering much pain."[51] The division commander, incredulous over the physician's lack of comprehension for his heinous actions, stated that "while the Brig. Gen. Comdg regrets extremely that a medical officer in this Division should be found so ignorant of his profession as to set up such a defense, he much prefers it to be so than to think any officer could be so grossly inhuman as to leave a wounded man to suffer."[52] Something that gave many white soldiers and officers pause, however, was the fact that if any incompetent or inhumane physician was in their ranks, they might eventually be the recipient of such inappropriate medical treatment themselves.

Because of prejudice and racism, obtaining physicians to serve for the USCT was often very difficult and obtaining competent physicians close to impossible. According to one surgeon regarding other physicians in the USCT, "You speak about the rank of surgeon. I have seen more confounded fools in the service with that rank that I care but little about it."[53]

The military hospitals in Washington, D.C., and the surrounding areas often contained upward of fifty thousand sick and wounded men. The types of injuries and maladies that men suffered, from abdominal wounds to head injuries and infections, were not to be believed, with typhoid and dysentery being the top contenders.[54]

An investigation of the Smallpox Hospital during the war by Albert Rogall found that the "colored soldiers in the Small Pox Hospital are neglected, that the rooms they occupy are unventilated and unclean."[55] On inspecting an African American hospital where his troops had been taken, Adjutant General Thomas was horrified: "Men were wearing the same clothing they had donned in the battle one month earlier, bloodstains and all, and had never changed them. One amputee complained that no one had bathed him and he still suffered from lice bites; another had no shirt because ten days earlier he had to discard it because of filth."[56] According to Thomas, "Had these been white soldiers, think you this would have been their condition? No."[57]

As stated earlier, the War Department had a difficult task in obtaining competent physicians to be part of the USCT. The surgeon general pushed for the formation of permanent boards to examine candidates who would be appointed as medical officers in the USCT in a number of large cities—Boston, New York, Washington, Philadelphia, Cincinnati and St. Louis—as well as temporary boards in various other locations.[58]

In addition to this, politicians often arranged deals through personal contact with some of the best medical schools in New York and New England to get the finest students into African American units in their district department. The Union army even arranged an early graduation program with selected medical schools for those students who agreed to enter the USCT immediately after successful completion of the college's oral examination and a written thesis. While these incentives helped increase the number of physicians treating African American soldiers, the military hierarchy struggled to obtain quality commanders and physicians for the USCT.

Burt Green Wilder was born in Boston in 1841. He entered Harvard at the age of eighteen, receiving his degree in 1862. Because Wilder had studied comparative anatomy, he was able to get an appointment as a medical cadet without attending medical school. Dr. Wilder was a medical cadet at the Judiciary Square Hospital in the Washington, D.C. Infantry in May 1863.[59]

> *Sunday, May 10th, 7:30 P.M. This morning came three letters from Surgeon General Dale, from Prof. Wyman, and from my father. The first offers me a position in the 55th Mass.; Wyman is rather non-committal but evidently does not advise my remaining here with no special chance for promotion; father is very desirous that I should accept. My chief reason for hesitating now is the needs of our wounded. Dr. Marsh does not like negroes and therefore does not advise me to go but he also says I ought not consider anything but my own advantage. I shall write Dr. Dale that I incline to accept.*[60]
>
> *May 23rd—I have been at the camp all the week and very hard at work, for recruits have been coming in fast. I have to examine them and am gaining quite a reputation for strictness, rejecting half a dozen that had been accepted by the surgeon specially sent to Buffalo. We have nearly 400 men now. Yesterday I organized the hospital. The hospital steward is a German who has had five years' experience in that capacity in the French army and seems well qualified. Whether he drinks or not remains to be seen. We have a cook, nurse, wardmaster and nine patients, some pretty sick. I have engaged a horse six years old from Mr. Gooding from Brookline; price 162.00.*[61]
>
> *Dr. Brown came in to borrow my artery forceps. Frank remarked, no one suits Dr. Brown, referring to a terrific scolding of the hospital cook for putting too much salt in the pea soup. Of course it was too salty for me, but as such things seldom happened I said nothing. Dr. Brown is really quite undignified sometimes in his language and I fear the men do not respect him as they should the surgeon of the regiment. Frank says he has heard them call him "that old crabbed," and make uncomplimentary comparisons between him and that "black whiskered young doctor." Their preference for me, however, gives me more to do, since they seldom apply to him for aid.*[62] *Sometimes I lose my patience with them either for their stupidity or because I think some are deceiving me as to the extent of their illness. Yesterday 200 reported themselves sick but this morning fewer and I cut down the excused ones to 140. It was a good occasion for a short but severe address to them on the folly and wickedness of such deception, wronging their comrades and me and their country; the good effect of my words was apparent in the demeanor and language of those who came to me afterward for advice and medicine.*[63]

My natural repugnance to medicine as a profession is lessening as I realize what an opportunity it offers for usefulness for helping others not only physically but morally, and for cheering the despondent. I may have to practice for some years until there offers a position in my chosen line; at present I am often and painfully conscious of my lack of regular medical training. Of practical surgery I saw so much in Washington that I feel fairly competent to deal with ordinary emergencies; but on the medical side I feel comparatively ignorant and I must study hard in order to justify my position and be equal to my probable responsibilities.[64]

Sunday, 13th, 3:30 PM. The early Sick Call is very objectionable in one respect; one would like to begin the day pleasantly but among the 150 to 175 men who report for treatment or excuse from duty are always a few whom I have reason to suspect of malingering; the effort to detect their frauds irritates me and sometimes, probably, renders me unjust to the really ill. When Dr. Babbitt arrives I hope he will perform this duty. The flies are greedy and undiscriminating; they will remain on a morsel till it actually enters the mouth, and they plunge headlong into ink and other unsuitable liquids; they can bite severely too.[65]

The early years of the Civil War were filled with frustration for Dr. Esther Hill Hawks, who desperately sought to contribute her medical skills to the Union cause. During the summer of 1861, she traveled to Washington, D.C., determined to serve as a doctor or, failing that, a nurse. When she discovered that the federal government was refusing to hire female doctors, she applied for a nursing position. Dorothea Dix, superintendent of Union army nurses, rejected Hawks's request. Hawks stayed on in Washington working as a volunteer in the army hospital. Her volunteer duties were limited to serving soldiers tea, coffee and snacks. She ended the war at the Freedmen's Bureau.

Many white doctors and nurses learned to greatly admire the African American soldiers in their care. According to author Stephen Oates in his book *A Woman of Valor: Clara Barton and the Civil War*, Clara Barton gained a great deal of respect for African American soldiers. On visiting General Hospital Number Ten for Colored Troops during the middle of the war, Barton's concern for and admiration of the African American troops was palpable: "As Clara moved from bed to bed, she showed a special concern for the black patients, touching their cheeks and soothing them with her soft musical voice."[66]

Louisa May Alcott, well known for authoring books such as *Little Women*, was a vital part of the Civil War medical family in Washington, D.C. On November 29, 1862, her thirtieth birthday, she volunteered to be a nurse in the capital. Her letters from her time in the war as a nurse led to her authoring the fictional

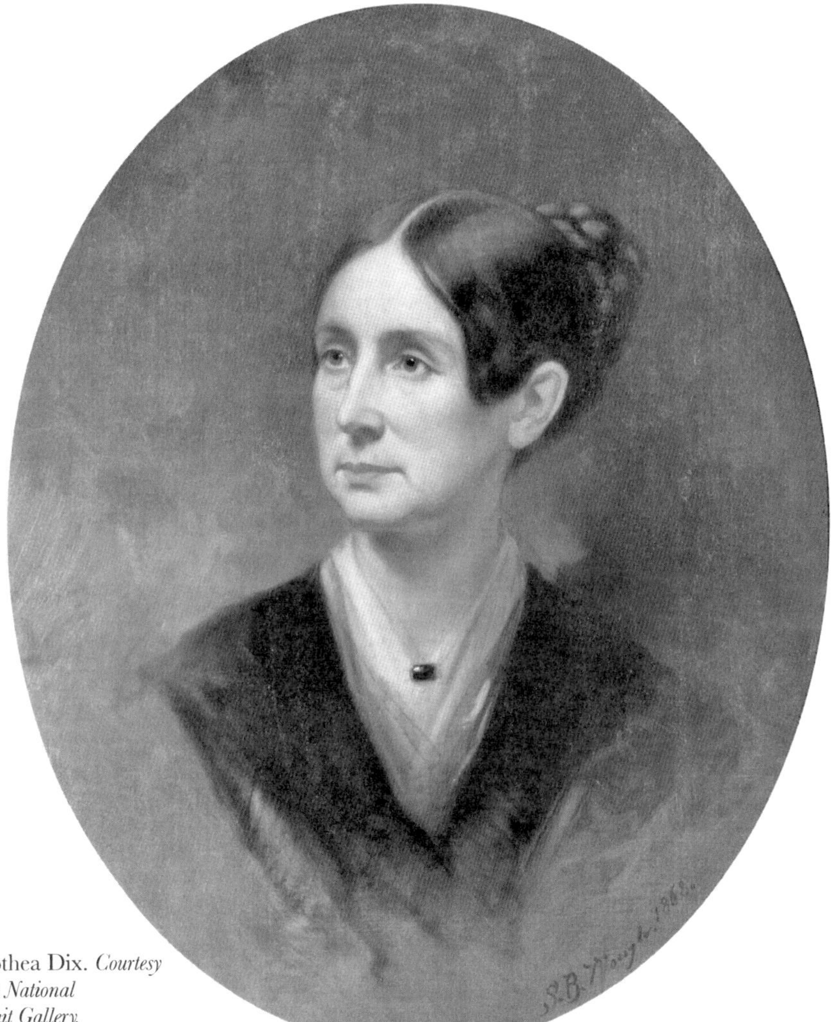

Dorothea Dix. *Courtesy of the National Portrait Gallery, Smithsonian Institution.*

book *Hospital Sketches*, in which she states, "The next hospital I enter will, I hope, be one for the colored regiments, as they seem to be providing their right to the admiration and kind offices of their white relations, who owe them so large a debt, a little part of which I shall be so proud to pay."[67]

At this point, the story of Nicholas Biddle, often referred to as the first casualty of the Civil War, deserves review. Biddle was born a slave in Delaware in the late 1790s. He escaped to Philadelphia and was servant to wealthy financier Nicholas Biddle, his namesake. Biddle eventually settled in Pottsville, Pennsylvania, in the

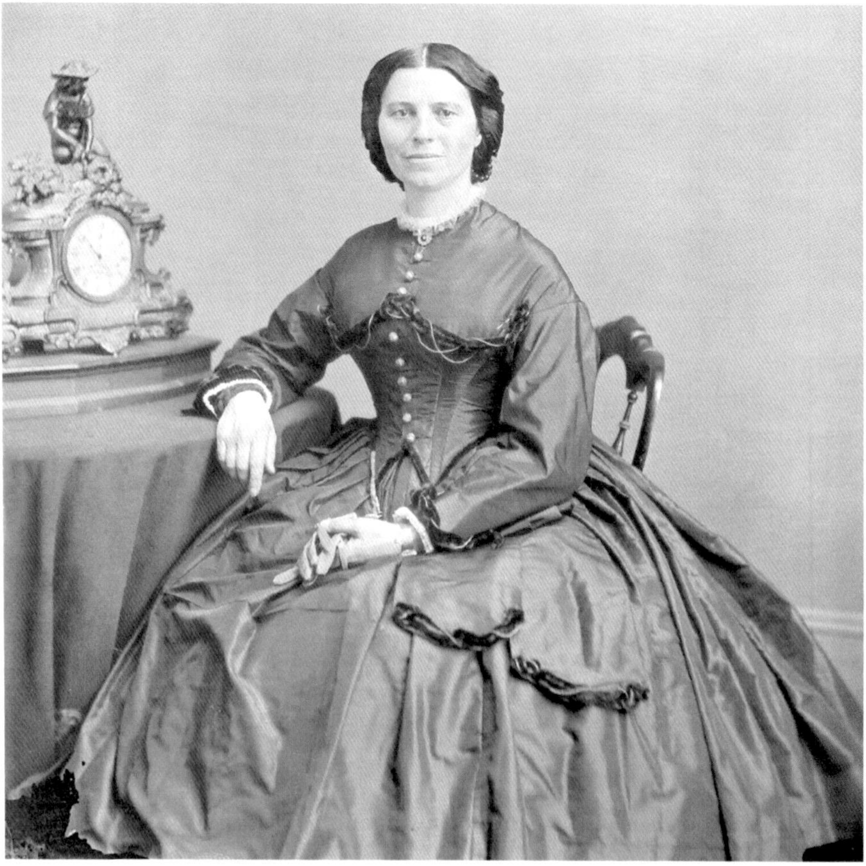

Clara Barton. *Courtesy of the United States National Archives and Records Administration.*

late 1850s/early 1860s doing various jobs, including street vending and selling oysters. The local militia were the Washington Artillerists, who Biddle became friendly with. Although African Americans were not allowed to be part of the militia, Biddle was given a uniform to wear. On April 15, 1861, President Lincoln called for 75,000 volunteers to serve for three months in the wake of the fall of Fort Sumter. The Washington Artillerists, with Biddle in uniform, answered the call. Biddle acted as an aide to the commanding officer. On the way to D.C., the company faced hostility. Biddle was injured quite seriously, taking a brick to his head. President Lincoln visited the soldiers, thanking them for making the dangerous journey. He greeted the soldiers, stating, "Officers and soldiers of the Washington Artillery…I did not come here to make a speech; the time for speechmaking has gone by, the time for action is at hand. I have come here to give you a warm welcome to the city of Washington, and to shake hands with every officer and soldier in your company providing you grant me the privilege." When Lincoln got to Biddle, he urged the man to seek additional treatment for his injury but Biddle insisted on remaining with the soldiers.

Biddle returned to Pottsville after his service, and he lived there until his death on August 2, 1876, at the age of eighty. Members of the Washington Artillerists and the National Light Infantry purchased a headstone for the impoverished Biddle that read, "In memory of Nicholas Biddle, died August 2, 1876, aged 80 years. His was the proud distinction of shedding the First Blood in the Late War for the Union, being wounded, while marching through Baltimore with the first Volunteers from Schuylkill County, 18, April 1861. Erected by his friends in Pottsville."[68]

In order to fully understand the plight of the wounded African American solider, it is instructive to get an overview of healthcare during that time. One of the best firsthand accounts comes from Walt Whitman, who served as a nurse during the war:

> *"Resolved" said a convention of free blacks, assembled at Poughkeepsie, New York, that summer to urge greater participation of black troops in the struggle for the Union. More effective remedies ought now to be many sleepless nights, how many women's tears, how many long and waking hours and days of suspense from every one of the Middle, Eastern and Western states have concentrated here? Our own New York, in the form of hundreds and thousands of her young men, may consider herself here; Pennsylvania, Ohio, Indiana, and all the West and Northwest the same, and all the New England States the same? Upon a few of these hospitals I have been almost daily calling on a mission, on my own account, for the sustenance and consolation of some of the most needy cases of sick and dying men for the last two months. One has much to learn to do good in these places. Great tact is required. These are not like other hospitals. By far the greatest proportion (I should say five-sixths) of the patients are American young men, intelligent of independent spirit, tender feelings used to a hardy and healthy life, largely the farmers are represented by their sons—largely the mechanics and workingmen of the cities. Then they are soldiers. All these points must be born in mind. People throughout northern cities have little or no idea of the great and prominent feature which these military hospitals and convalescent camps make in and around Washington. There are not merely two or three or a dozen, but some fifty of them of different degrees of capacity. Some have a thousand and more patients. The newspapers here find it necessary to print every day a directory of the hospitals—a long list something like what a directory of the*

> *churches would be New York, Philadelphia, or Boston. The government which really tries, I think to do the best and quickest it can for these sad necessities is gradually settling down to adopt the plan of placing the hospitals in clusters of one-story wooden barracks with their accompanying tents and sheds for cooking and all needed purposes. Taking all things into consideration, no doubt these are best adapted to the purpose, better than using churches and large public buildings like the Patent Office. These sheds now adopted are long, one-story edifices, sometimes ranged along in a row with their heads to the street, and numbered either alphabetically—Wards A or B, C, D, and so on; or Wards 1, 2, 3, etc. The middle one will be marked by a flagstaff, and is the office of the establishment, with rooms for the ward surgeons, etc. One of these sheds or wards will contain sixty cots; sometimes, on an emergency, they move them close together and crowd in more. Some of the barracks are larger, with of course more inmates. Frequently there are tents—more comfortable here than one might think—whatever they may be down in the army. Each ward has a ward-mater and generally a nurse for every ten or twelve men. A ward surgeon has, generally, two wards, although this varies. Some of the wards have a woman nurse; the Armory-Square wards have some very good ones. The one in Ward E is one of the best. A few weeks ago the vast area of the second story of that noblest of Washington building—the Patent Office—was crowded close with rows of the sick, badly wounded and dying soldiers. They were placed in three very large apartments. I went there several times. It was a strange, solemn, and—with all its features of suffering and death—a sort of fascinating sight. Some, I found, needed a little cheering up and friendly consolation at that time, for they went to sleep better afterwards.*[69] *There are plenty of excellent clean old black women that would make tiptop nurses.*[70] *There are getting to be many black troops. There is one very good regiment here; black as tar; they go around have the regular uniform, they submit to no nonsense. Others are constantly forming. It is getting to be common sight.*[71]

Healthcare of African American Soldiers During the Civil War

When Governor Andrew queried Secretary of War Stanton as to whether there could also be the appointment of African American company officers, assistant surgeons and a chaplain, Stanton indicated that this was an open question for Congress and the president. Even once certain flexibility was

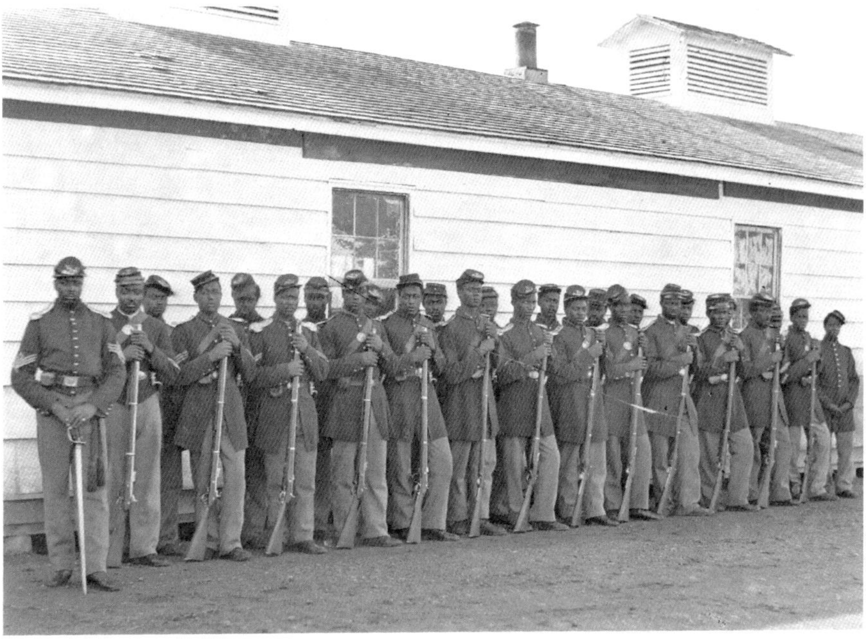

Company E of the Fourth Regiment of the United States Colored Troops. *Courtesy of the Library of Congress, Washington, D.C.*

given with respect to raising regiments with African American officers, the possibility of African Americans rising in the ranks was quite dismal indeed. Yet thirty-two African American men in total received appointments in the USCT and fourteen of these were chaplains.[72]

On the antislavery front, abolitionists knew that having African American soldiers in the Union army would be the way to truly ensure equality for all. In 1862, Congress authorized recruitment of African American regiments, but it wasn't until 1863 that regiments actually began to be formed.

While, at the beginning of the war, slaves made their way to D.C. in order to escape the chains of slavery, as the Union army moved farther and farther into Confederate territory, slaves had the opportunity of escaping to the Northern lines. While Union troops might have had their own opinions about slaves, they did nothing to stop them from crossing lines in order to gain their freedom from slavery.[73] However, while Union troops did not stop slaves from crossing Union lines, the thought of ex-slaves serving in the Union army was an entirely different matter altogether. There were several reports after Bull Run about the formation of regiments of African American troops. While President Lincoln

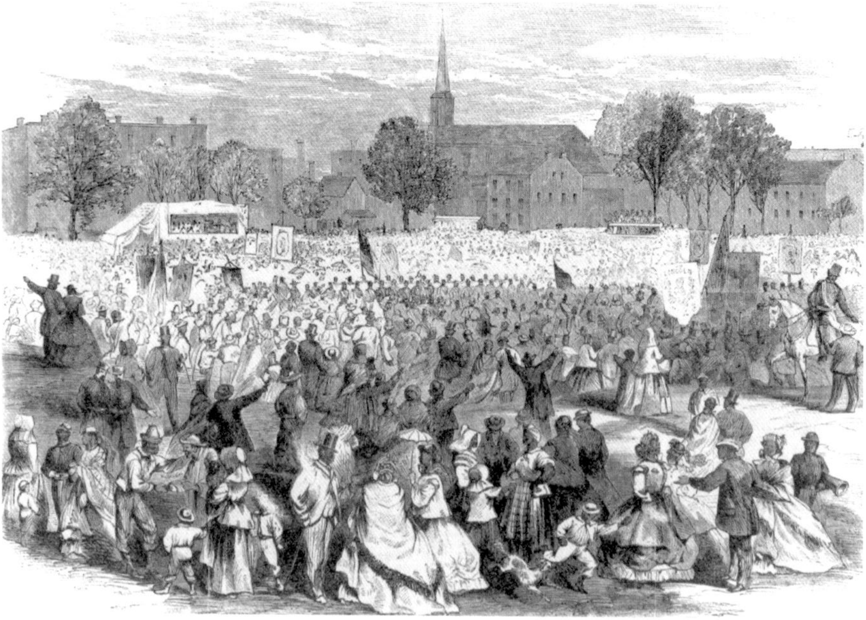

Celebration of the abolition of slavery in Washington, D.C. *Courtesy of the Library of Congress, Washington, D.C.*

Opposite: The Emancipation Proclamation. *Courtesy of the Library of Congress, Washington, D.C.*

took time to decide on the matter, abolitionists in the North voiced strong opinions regarding ex-slaves fighting for their country and freedom. From local abolitionists in Boston to politicians such as Charles Sumner, the notion of African Americans fighting for the Union was taking shape.[74]

While the issue of African Americans either fighting in the Union army or serving in some capacity continued, the casualties and injuries on the Union side continued to grow. With almost one million African Americans—free men and slaves—being of age to fight in the war, their possible contribution to the effort could no longer be ignored. With the issuing of the Emancipation Proclamation, former slaves were invited into the ranks of the armed forces.

Not all Union soldiers or officers were pleased with this turn of events, with General William T. Sherman as one of the more vocal opponents. "I thought a soldier was to be an active machine, a fighter,"[75] he told his brother John, a United States senator from Ohio. "Dirt or cotton will stop a bullet better than a man's body." According to Sherman, "I have no confidence in [African Americans] and don't want them mixed up with our white soldiers."[76] Beyond

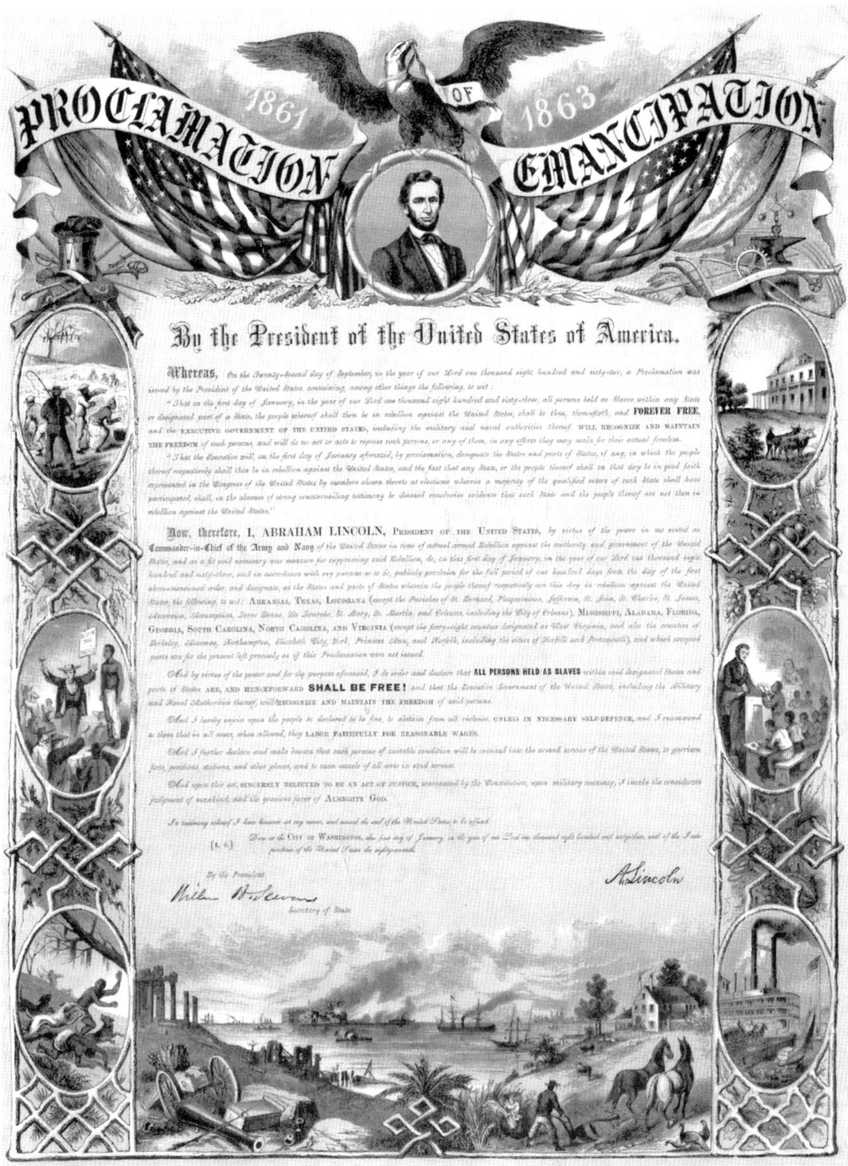

prejudices that Sherman had, as a military man, a larger concern was probably the logistics of forming new regiments and what that would mean to the war effort. "All who deal with troops in fact instead of theory," he told Grant, "know that the knowledge of the little details of Camp Life is absolutely necessary to keep men alive. New Regiments for want of this knowledge have measles, mumps, diarrhea and the whole catalogue of infantile diseases."[77]

Another point that abolitionists were probably reluctant to acknowledge but that Sherman was fully aware of was, given the history many ex-slaves had with this country, how many of them were interested in picking up arms and giving their lives to fight for it? This would become apparent over the course of the war, but in the beginning of 1863, it was an open question.

The USCT was organized in regiments that represented the three branches of the army: cavalry, artillery and infantry. It grew to include seven regiments of cavalry, more than a dozen of artillery and well over one hundred of infantry.[78] One of the more noted D.C. regiments was the Fourth Regiment. The regiment was organized in Baltimore from July 15 to September 1, 1863. Three members of the regiment received the Medal of Honor: Christian Fleetwood, Alfred Hilton and Charles Veale. The regiment saw action in various parts of the country but was affiliated with the Washington, D.C. area. Private James Slaughter was a member of the regiment from September 1863 until January 1865.[79]

Medal of Honor–winner Christian Fleetwood was born in Baltimore in 1840. He enlisted in the regiment in August 1863 as a sergeant and was quickly promoted to sergeant major. Following his service, he was honorably discharged in 1866. He settled in Washington, D.C., and worked for the government as a battalion commander with the D.C. National Guard. He died of heart failure on September 28, 1914, at the age of seventy-four.[80]

Enlisting African Americans in the Union army was complicated on multiple levels, including interest on the parts of Northerners, abolitionists and the ex-slaves themselves. In a famous quote, Lincoln stated, "If I could save the Union without freeing a slave, I would do it and if I could save it by freeing some and leaving others alone I would also do that."[81] Lincoln had many groups to appease and had to consider the issue of border state sentiment, European support and the reconstitution of the country as a whole. But finally, with the Battle of Antietam as a backdrop, Lincoln put forth the Emancipation Proclamation.[82]

Later in the war, Washington, D.C. army camps would be a source of recruitment, healthcare and services. The government began to organize camps to provide shelter on Capitol Hill, the Camp Barker area, the U Street Corridor and even Freedmen's Village in Arlington County. They also had clergy, healthcare providers and others giving care to those in the camps.[83]

The conditions for contrabands in Washington, D.C., were often less than ideal. According to Harriet Jacobs, a reporter for the *Liberator*:

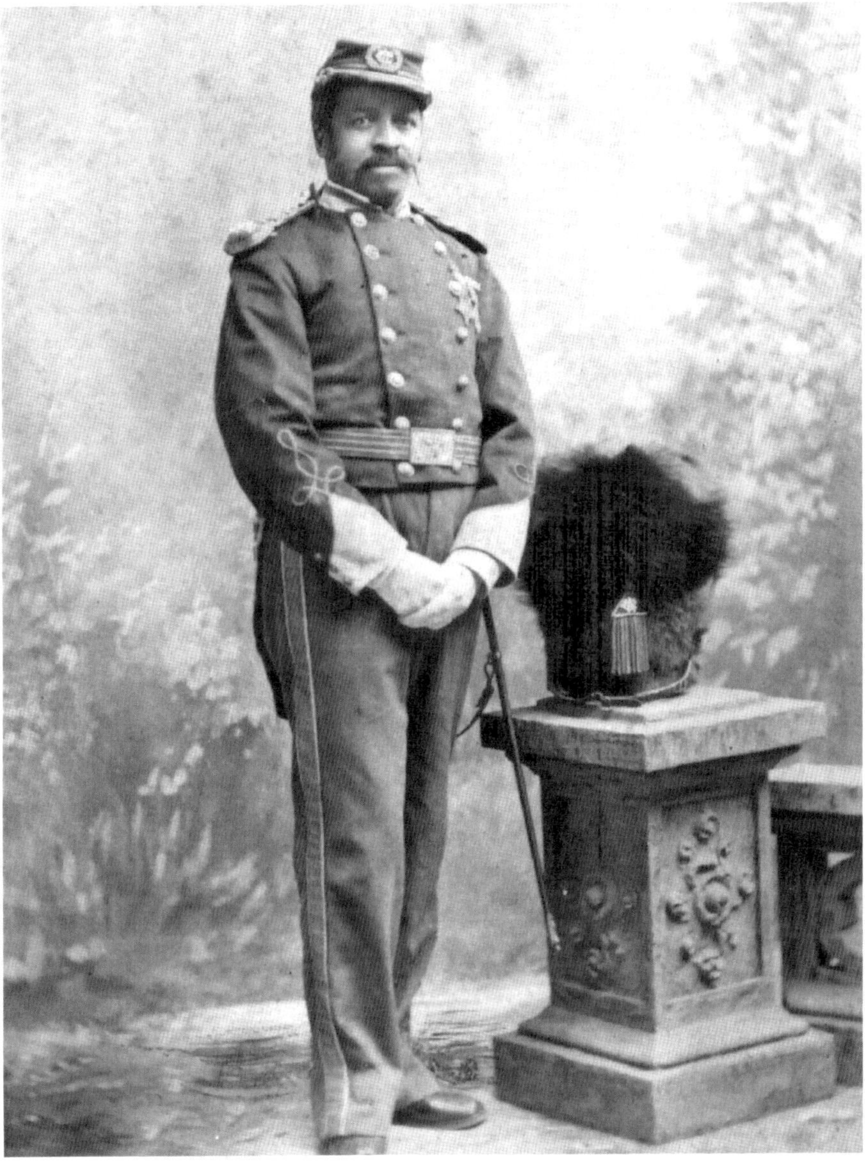

Sergeant Major Christian Fleetwood. *Courtesy of the Library of Congress, Washington, D.C.*

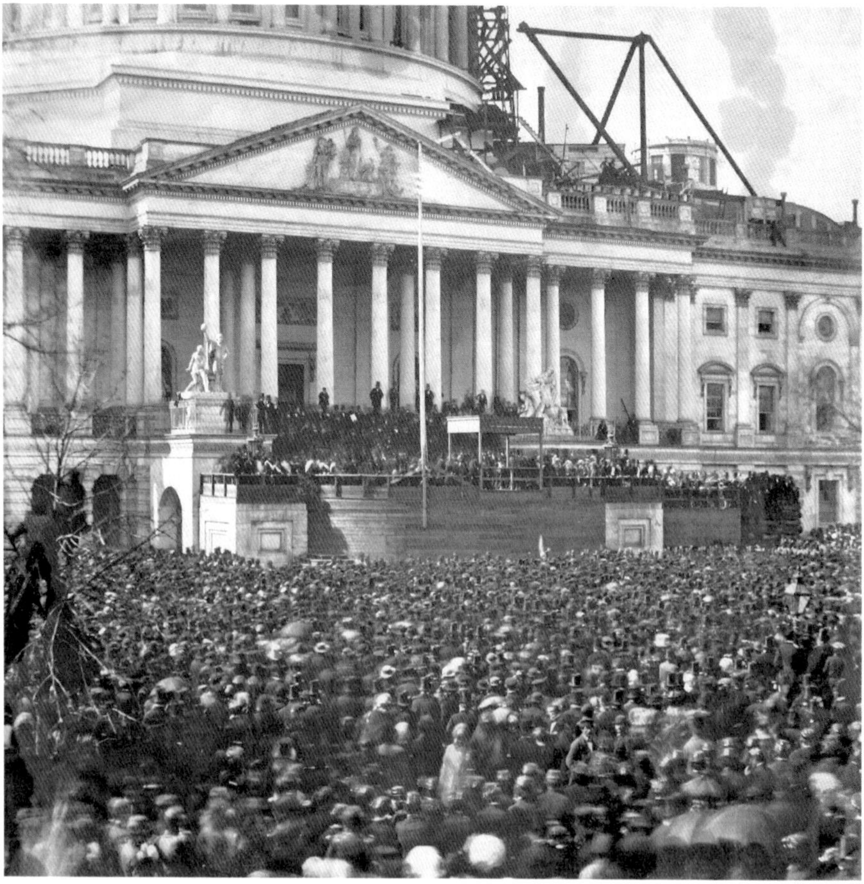

President Abraham Lincoln's first inauguration, 1861. *Courtesy of the Library of Congress, Washington, D.C.*

> *I went to Duff Green's Row, government headquarters for the contrabands here. I found men, women and children all huddled together without any distinction of regard to age or sex, some of them were in the most pitiable condition. Many were sick with measles, diphtheria, scarlet or typhoid fever. Some had a few filthy rags to lie on, others had nothing but the bare floor for a couch…Some of them have been so degraded by slavery that they do not know the usages of civilized life: they know little else than the handle of the hoe, the plough, the cotton pad and the overseer's lash.*

According to author John David Smith:

> *Army recruiters had indeed promised black enlistees fair and equal treatment…Throughout their service, black soldiers received discriminatory duties, inferior assignments, inadequate care, insufficient training, and insults from white soldiers.*[84]

According to author James McPherson:

> *Although partly remedied in 1864, the inequality of pay was only one of several signs that black regiments were considered second-class soldiers. Some regiments functioned initially as labor battalions to dig trenches, load and unload supplies, and perform heavy fatigue duty for white troops. Even when organized in combat units, black soldiers often carried inferior arms and equipment. Lincoln originally planned to use black troops to garrison forts, protect supply dumps and wagon trains, and perform rear-area duties thereby releasing white regiments for front-line operations. Three considerations underlay this: (1) skepticism about whether African Americans would make good combat soldiers; (2) a belief that freemen were better acclimated to garrison duty in the deep South, where northern soldiers suffered much sickness; and (3) the fact that rear-area duties would reduce the possibility of capture.*[85]

According to Chulhee Lee:

> *Even after black men were officially mustered in the army, they were discriminated against in various ways. Black recruits were not permitted to become commissioned officers, and were paid much less than white soldiers of their same rank. Furthermore, they were much more likely to be assigned to heavy manual duties while white soldiers were sent to fight in the battlegrounds.*[86]

After battle, many of the African American soldiers were put back on fatigue duty—pitching tents and other menial labor. Because of this hard work, much of these soldiers' clothing was in rags, with some African American soldiers actually owing the government money.[87]

The dress of African American regiments was a source of great study. How regiments were dressed varied greatly. While some of the regiments were extremely well dressed, others were not so. Some of the soldiers were dressed in short sleeves and had no shoes. There was a clear explanation for much of this and its roots lay in fatigue duty. An inordinate amount of fatigue

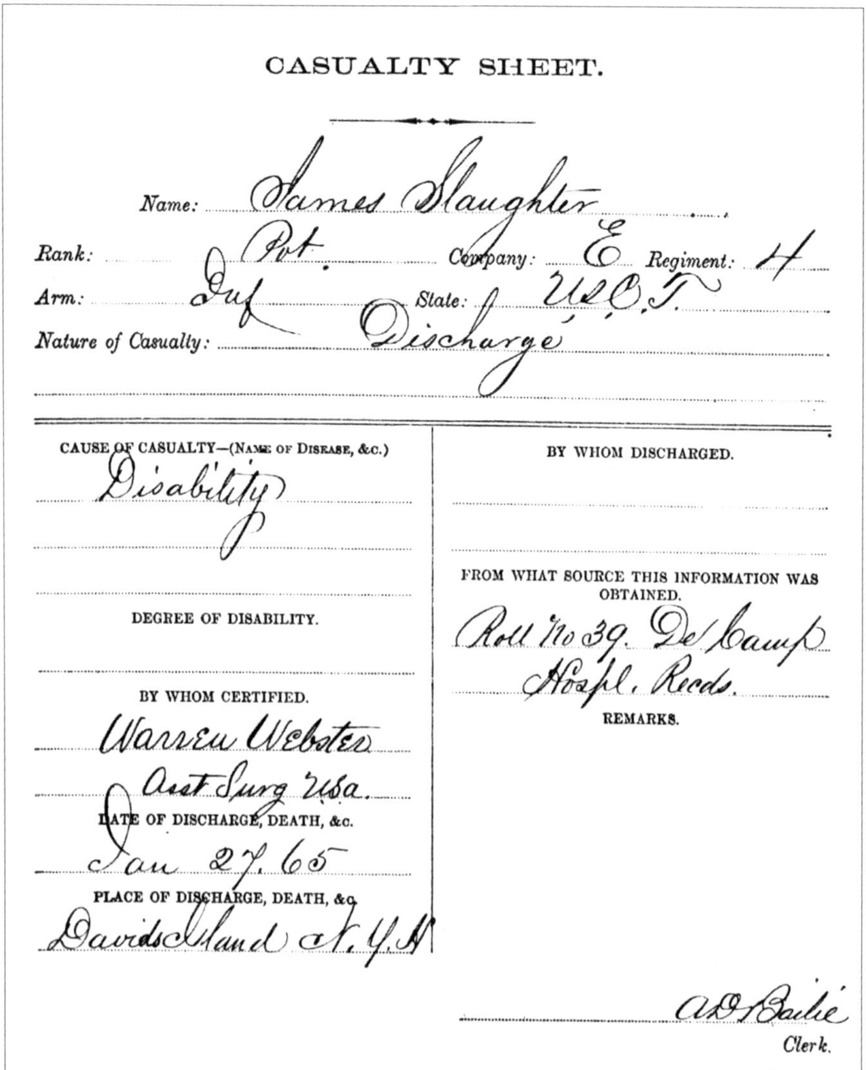

CASUALTY SHEET.

Name: James Slaughter

Rank: Pvt. Company: E Regiment: 4

Arm: Inf State: U.S.C.T.

Nature of Casualty: Discharge

CAUSE OF CASUALTY—(NAME OF DISEASE, &c.)

Disability

DEGREE OF DISABILITY.

BY WHOM CERTIFIED.

Warren Webster

Asst Surg USA.

DATE OF DISCHARGE, DEATH, &c.

Jan 27. 65

PLACE OF DISCHARGE, DEATH, &c.

Davids Island N.Y.H

BY WHOM DISCHARGED.

FROM WHAT SOURCE THIS INFORMATION WAS OBTAINED.

Roll No 39. De Camp Hospl. Records.

REMARKS.

A D Bailie

Clerk.

(170)

Records of Private James Slaughter, Company E of the Fourth Regiment. *Courtesy of the United States National Archives and Records Administration.*

and guard duty made it extremely difficult for African Americans to have the kind of time that was necessary to keep uniforms and equipment well maintained. When the soldiers did have the time to care for their uniforms, it was a way for them to shine.[88]

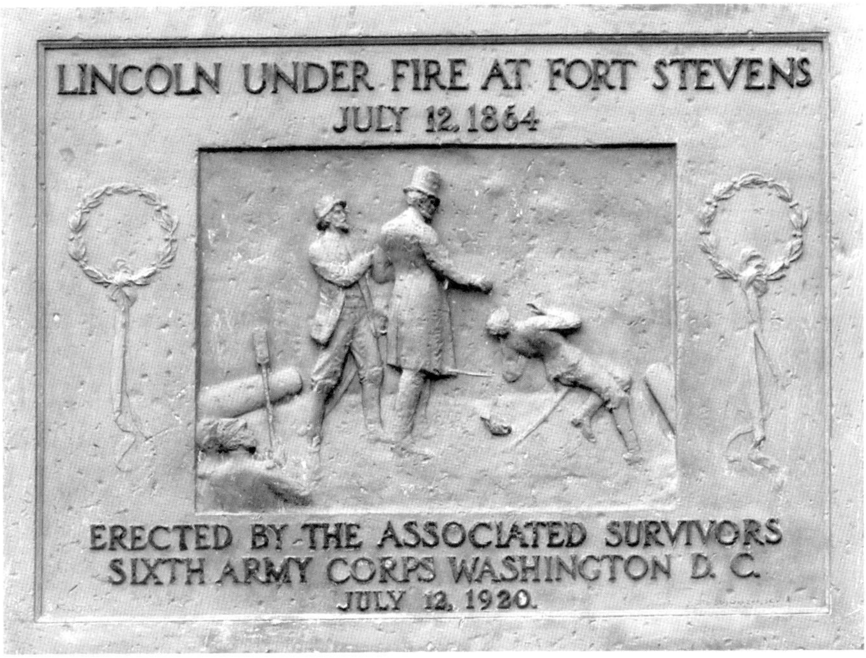
LINCOLN UNDER FIRE AT FORT STEVENS
JULY 12, 1864
ERECTED BY THE ASSOCIATED SURVIVORS
SIXTH ARMY CORPS WASHINGTON D.C.
JULY 12, 1920.

A remembrance of Abraham Lincoln's visit to Fort Stevens. *Courtesy of Wikimedia Commons.*

While most African Americans served in the war effort as soldiers, there were a variety of other roles that they also filled, including healthcare workers, wagoners, cooks and teamsters. Other than the healthcare workers, these individuals were often still referred to as soldiers, and in white regiments, if they were serving in these capacities, they were included in the regiment's fatalities rather than those of the USCT. Therefore, casualty numbers for the African American regiments were skewed because they were not factored into numbers for the African American regiments.[89]

On August 8, 1862, General Sherman ordered African Americans to be used for the war effort but not in the role of soldiers. The thought was that they could be utilized in other capacities, such as company cooks, laborers and nurses.[90] Based on this, Congress passed an act specifying the composition of regiments. For every regiment of up to thirty men, there was to be one cook provided. Two cooks were required for companies over thirty men. Furthermore, with respect to compensation, these individuals were to receive ten dollars per month with three dollars of that pay in clothing. This was the same compensation for African American soldiers.[91]

General Grant also allowed the hiring of African Americans for various services and authorized, in his Department of the Tennessee, the use within each of his regiments and companies of one African American cook per fifteen men and one African American teamster for every wagon.[92] The First USCT, formed in D.C., initially had difficulty filling its ranks due to the fact that a large number of African Americans in D.C. were already employed as laborers and teamsters and were secure in these vocations. Additionally, African Americans residing in D.C. who decided to join regiments such as the First USCT had to contend with being accosted and assaulted on the streets of the city when in uniform. Nevertheless, despite these setbacks, numbers for African American regiments increased, with the First USCT numbering ten companies of almost seven hundred men each.[93]

According to the historian Aptheker:

> *For a regular* [army] *company, the two undercooks will be enlisted; for a volunteer company they will be mustered into service, as in the case of other soldiers. In each case a remark will be made on their enlistment papers showing that they are undercooks of African descent. Their names will be borne on the company muster rolls at the foot of the list of privates. They will be paid, and their accounts will be kept, like other enlisted men.* [That is, the manner of payment was to be identical, not the sum disbursed.] *They will also be discharged in the same manner as other soldiers.*[94]

While African American undercooks were enlisted in regiments prior to this War Department order, there were some distinct discrepancies in how the enlistments were handled. The notion was that African Americans who served in this capacity would be treated as though they were soldiers, albeit receiving a lower wage than white soldiers. But theory did not always live up to practice.[95]

African Americans in capacities other than fighting had enlistment papers that looked remarkably similar to those of their white counterparts, thus making it difficult to distinguish the African American non-fighting soldiers from other white soldiers in the armed services. They also appeared to have similar uniforms to their white counterparts.

Aptheker says:

> *It appears safe to say that at least as many African Americans were hired by the Government as were formally enrolled in its Army's ranks; that is to say, something like 200,000 or 250,000 men and women, by their labor and other activities, under the direct supervision of Government agencies, helped bring the Civil War to a successful end.*[96]

Many nonenlisted African Americans were used in military roles that brought them into proximity with the actual battleground and certainly into day-to-day relationships with other soldiers. One such type of employment, undertaken by several thousand African Americans, was that as a servant or orderly for officers. African Americans appear to have served in the role of servant for the entire length of the war. It also appears that some of these men were taken as prisoners of war.

Apthekar continues:

> *That these servants were involved in all the trials of war is clear. Thus, four* [African American] *orderlies were among the 403 Federal prisoners of war delivered to Fort Monroe on February 20, 1862 by Confederate exchange officers. Three days later, 372 Federal prisoners of war arrived, in exchange, at the same place, and among them were ten* [African Americans], *probably, but not certainly, officers' servants.*[97]

Another story of a possible African American scout finds its roots in the life of Tomi Heath who, in early 1864 was arrested by Confederate forces for having "acted as a guide to the enemy," but the district attorney felt sufficient evidence to convict for treason was not available. He noted the recent suspension of the writ of habeas corpus and recommended that the secretary of war order Heath's incarceration without trial. He did this because "the crime with which he is charged is one of such frequent occurrence that an example should be made of Heath. It is a matter of notoriety in the sections of the Confederacy where raids are frequent that the guides of the enemy are nearly always free African Americans and slaves."[98]

Possibly as many as fifty African American volunteers were kept constantly employed in the important duties of spies, scouts and guides. In these lines of work, they were invaluable to the Union army. They frequently went from thirty to three hundred miles within the enemy's lines, visiting enemy camps and bringing back vital information. Often on these errands, they barely escaped with their lives. Two or three of them were taken prisoner; one of these was known to have been shot, and the fates of the others were not ascertained.[99]

From chopping down trees to improving roads and preparing gun positions, African American soldiers were instrumental in constructing the surroundings within which all soldiers fought. African Americans who performed these duties were paid in the same manner as other African Americans who were part of the Union's forces.[100]

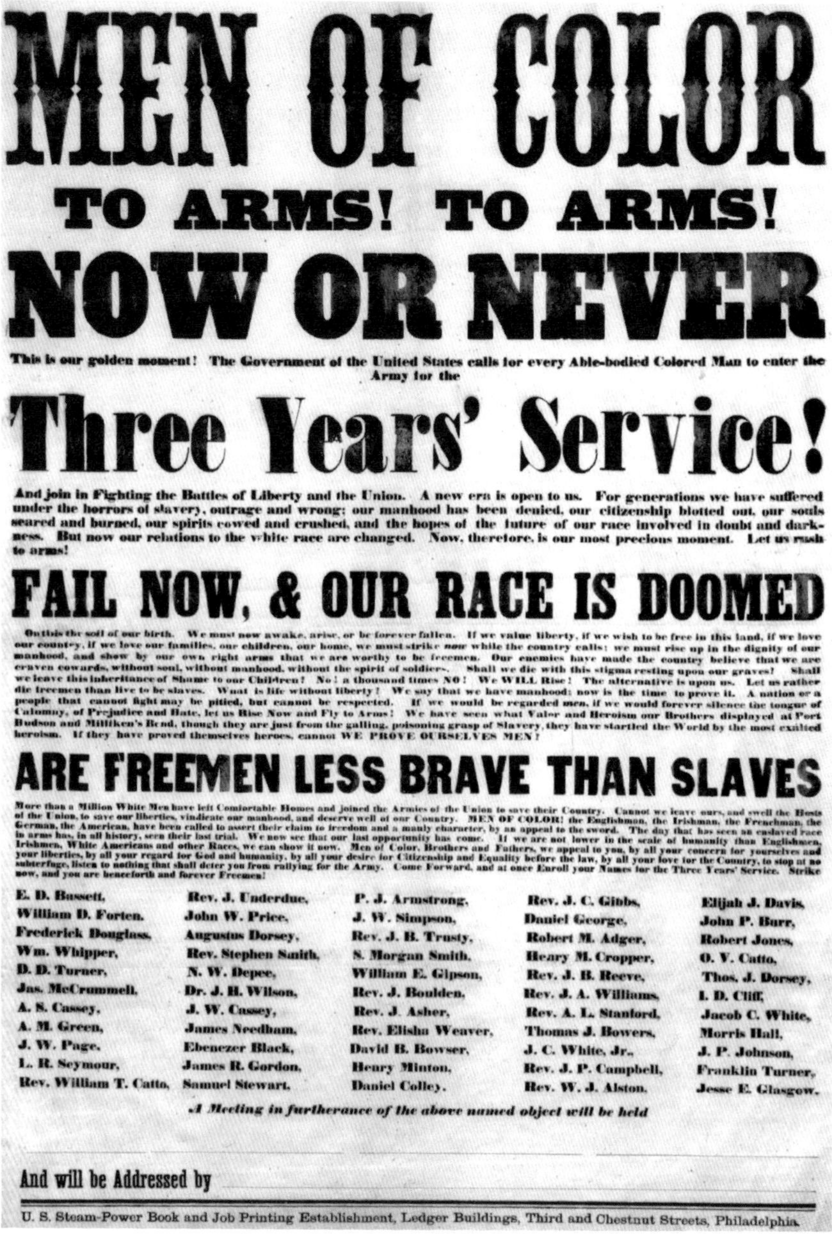

MEN OF COLOR

TO ARMS! TO ARMS!

NOW OR NEVER

This is our golden moment! The Government of the United States calls for every Able-bodied Colored Man to enter the Army for the

Three Years' Service!

And join in Fighting the Battles of Liberty and the Union. A new era is open to us. For generations we have suffered under the horrors of slavery, outrage and wrong; our manhood has been denied, our citizenship blotted out, our souls seared and burned, our spirits cowed and crushed, and the hopes of the future of our race involved in doubt and darkness. But now our relations to the white race are changed. Now, therefore, is our most precious moment. Let us rush to arms!

FAIL NOW, & OUR RACE IS DOOMED

On this the soil of our birth. We must now awake, arise, or be forever fallen. If we value liberty, if we wish to be free in this land, if we love our country, if we love our families, our children, our home, we must strike *now* while the country calls: we must rise up in the dignity of our manhood, and show by our own right arms that we are worthy to be freemen. Our enemies have made the country believe that we are craven cowards, without soul, without manhood, without the spirit of soldiers. Shall we die with this stigma resting upon our graves? Shall we leave this inheritance of Shame to our Children? No! a thousand times NO! We WILL Rise! The alternative is upon us. Let us rather die freemen than live to be slaves. What is life without liberty? We say that we have manhood; now is the time to prove it. A nation or a people that cannot fight may be pitied, but cannot be respected. If we would be regarded *men*, if we would forever silence the tongue of Calumny, of Prejudice and Hate, let us Rise Now and Fly to Arms! We have seen what Valor and Heroism our Brothers displayed at Port Hudson and Milliken's Bend, though they are just from the galling, poisoning grasp of Slavery, they have startled the World by the most exalted heroism. If they have proved themselves heroes, cannot WE PROVE OURSELVES MEN?

ARE FREEMEN LESS BRAVE THAN SLAVES

More than a Million White Men have left Comfortable Homes and joined the Armies of the Union to save their Country. Cannot we leave ours, and swell the Hosts of the Union, to save our liberties, vindicate our manhood, and deserve well of our Country. MEN OF COLOR! the Englishman, the Irishman, the Frenchman, the German, the American, have been called to assert their claim to freedom and a manly character, by an appeal to the sword. The day that has seen an enslaved race in arms has, in all history, seen their last trial. We now see that our last opportunity has come. If we are not lower in the scale of humanity than Englishmen, Irishmen, White Americans and other Races, we can show it now. *Men of Color, Brothers and Fathers*, we appeal to you, by all your concern for yourselves and your liberties, by all your regard for God and humanity, by all your desire for Citizenship and Equality before the law, by all your love for the Country, to stop at no subterfuge, listen to nothing that shall deter you from rallying for the Army. Come Forward, and at once Enroll your Names for the Three Years' Service. Strike now, and you are henceforth and forever Freemen!

E. D. Bassett,
William D. Forten,
Frederick Douglass,
Wm. Whipper,
D. D. Turner,
Jas. McCrummell,
A. S. Cassey,
A. M. Green,
J. W. Page,
L. R. Seymour,
Rev. William T. Catto,
Rev. J. Underdue,
John W. Price,
Augustus Dorsey,
Rev. Stephen Smith,
N. W. Depee,
Dr. J. H. Wilson,
J. W. Cassey,
James Needham,
Ebenezer Black,
James R. Gordon,
Samuel Stewart,
P. J. Armstrong,
J. W. Simpson,
Rev. J. B. Trusty,
S. Morgan Smith,
William E. Gipson,
Rev. J. Boulden,
Rev. J. Asher,
Rev. Elisha Weaver,
David B. Bowser,
Henry Minton,
Daniel Colley,
Rev. J. C. Gibbs,
Daniel George,
Robert M. Adger,
Henry M. Cropper,
Rev. J. B. Reeve,
Rev. J. A. Williams,
Rev. A. L. Stanford,
Thomas J. Bowers,
J. C. White, Jr.,
Rev. J. P. Campbell,
Rev. W. J. Alston,
Elijah J. Davis,
John P. Burr,
Robert Jones,
O. V. Catto,
Thos. J. Dorsey,
I. D. Cliff,
Jacob C. White,
Morris Hall,
J. P. Johnson,
Franklin Turner,
Jesse E. Glasgow.

A Meeting in furtherance of the above named object will be held

And will be Addressed by

U. S. Steam-Power Book and Job Printing Establishment, Ledger Buildings, Third and Chestnut Streets, Philadelphia.

Men of color at arms. *Courtesy of the Gilder Lehrman Institute of American History.*

African American soldiers, as much as they wanted to be in the mainstream, wound up digging trenches and performing other menial labor more than their white counterparts. The type of work African American troops engaged in led to higher incidents of injuries relative to other soldiers. Many who supported African American soldiers being a part of the war effort believed that those soldiers would be seeing active combat, but there was a movement afoot to ensure that African American soldiers saw little to no actual combat. In fact, it was a common belief that African American troops were more suited to perform hard labor tasks than to perform soldiers' duties. Much of this labor was relentless and difficult. From working in sweltering heat to "fatigue labor," African American soldiers were expected to work under grueling conditions for long periods of time, not unlike what some had experienced before the war.[101]

This created an odd cycle in which the white soldiers assigned menial tasks to the African American soldiers and then deemed them to be inferior to the white soldiers because they performed such tasks.

Such work had physical and healthcare implications for the soldiers. According to historian John David Smith, while 67,178 of the African American soldiers who served in the army died, a mere 2,751 were killed in combat, with the rest dying from wounds or disease. The African American soldiers' illnesses were made fatal by the poor health they suffered due to overwork.[102] The level of fatigue duty also affected morale and the psyche. It was long, arduous work.[103]

From the beginning of the Civil War, the utilization of African American soldiers was essentially decided on a case-by-case basis within each regiment. White officers and soldiers did not always trust African American soldiers. In fact, many white officers believed that if they used African American soldiers, it should be only as laborers, servants and cooks.[104]

General Sherman, for example, was in great favor of using African Americans as laborers. In fact, he reported to the adjutant general, "I have used [African American soldiers] with great success."[105]

Payday was wonderful for soldiers. In addition to having funds to send to loved ones, soldiers were able to indulge in treats for themselves that made the work go somewhat faster. From fresh fruits and foods to getting additional provisions and simply being able to spend time with comrades in a relaxed fashion, leisure time for the soldiers was welcome indeed.[106]

The whole concept behind the employment of African American troops by the Union army goes far in explaining their excessive mortality rates.

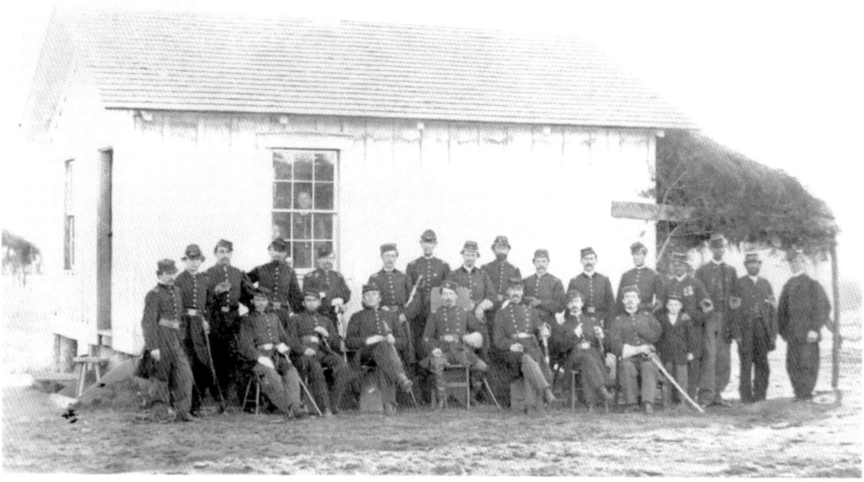

Officers of the Fourth Colored Infantry. *Courtesy of the Library of Congress, Washington, D.C.*

The ambivalence of the federal government in employing African American soldiers is telling. The wording of the law that passed on July 17, 1862, by which Congress finally authorized the president to employ African American troops, is significant. Under this document, the president might, if he wished, receive African Americans into the armed services for various purposes, including performing camp service or labor in both the military and naval services.

On the other hand, the general in chief of the Federal army, Major General Halleck, hearing some nine months later of a reluctance among certain officers in General Grant's command to utilize African Americans, wrote to Grant, unofficially, that the government now was committed to their use, particularly "as a military force for the defense of forts, depots…if they can be used to hold points on the Mississippi during the sickly season, it will afford much relief to our armies." The divergence in the thinking of the commanding officers and "our armies" is noteworthy.[107]

According to the commissioner for the Organization of Colored Troops, "The colored men here are treated like brutes; any officer who wants them, I am told, impresses on his own authority; and it is seldom that they are paid." Ordinary citizens also noticed the manner in which troops were treated and regarded it with disdain.[108]

On November 25, 1863, General Order No. 105 was issued, calling attention to the fact that African American troops were taking on an inordinate amount of fatigue duty, to their own detriment: "Colored troops will not be required to perform any labor which is not shared by the white troops, but will receive, in all respects...the same opportunities for drill and instructions."[109]

While African Americans fought in countless battles during the war, generals like Sherman were never proponents of utilizing African Americans in the war. Sherman stated, "I believe the African Americans better serve the army as teamsters, pioneers and servants…I must have labor and a large quantity of it. I confess I would prefer three hundred (300) African Americans armed with spades and axes than a thousand as soldiers."[110] Sherman was not alone in his thoughts regarding African American soldiers. The fatigue work that African American soldiers engaged in is legendary, and African Americans as well as their commanders had to fight in order to engage in battle with their white counterparts. In an odd turn, because African Americans were not automatically placed in combat situations, they were viewed by their white counterparts as not combat ready for purposes of provisions. From worn-out shoes and clothes to inferior food and drilling without real or adequate rifles, these soldiers received subpar supplies with the excuse that they were not doing the type of battle that white soldiers were engaged in. Medical care for African American soldiers was also inadequate, and as is clear in Civil War Washington, D.C., their hospitals lacked proper medicines and provisions.[111]

The question of what to do with the African American soldier would haunt military commanders and politicians throughout the war. This was especially true for commanders in and around Washington, D.C., where the safety of the capital depended on such decisions. On the one hand, there were abolitionists and supporters, such as Governor Andrew of Massachusetts, who firmly believed in the right and need of African Americans to fight for their country. On the other hand, there were generals, such as Sherman, who did not trust African Americans taking up arms: "Is not an African American as good as a white man to stop a bullet? Yes and a sand bag is better but can an African American do our skirmishing and picket duty? Can they improvise bridges, sorties, flank movements, etc. like the white man can? I say no."[112]

Sherman's friend General Grant said, "Yes, I have given the subject of arming the African Americans my hearty support. This with the emancipation of the African Americans is the heaviest blow yet given the Confederacy…By arming the African American we have added a powerful ally. They will make good soldiers and taking them from the enemy weakens him in the same proportion they strengthen us."[113] From D.C., Lincoln had come to agree with Grant, and when the opposition complained, he hit back hard.

The casualty rates during the war for African American soldiers were high.[114] There were a number of contributing factors to this. Many African American troops had no previous exposure to diseases that were rampant in military camps, yet military authorities assigned African American commands to unhealthy sites to do manual labor. Military personnel assumed African Americans were immune to all tropical diseases. African Americans were also thought to be mentally inferior to whites, and this also contributed to the physical and psychological problems faced by these troops.[115]

There were four regiments of African Americans that were technically not part of the USCT. While the injury and death rates for these regiments are usually added to the numbers for the USCT overall, they are sometimes also attributed to the states in which these regiments were raised.[116] The regiments were the Twenty-ninth Regiment of Connecticut Volunteer Infantry, the Fifth Regiment of Massachusetts Cavalry and the Fifty-fourth and Fifty-fifth Regiments of Massachusetts Volunteer Infantry.[117] Furthermore, there were some African American regiments raised for brief amounts of time but again, those numbers would not be included in the USCT overall numbers.[118]

Many white soldiers and officers assumed that African Americans should do what amounted to the "dirty work" of the war, including digging trenches and wells and pitching tents.[119] Having African American soldiers constantly perform such physically tolling manual labor was psychologically and physically exhausting for them.[120] According to historian James McPherson:

> *The substitution of black for white troops in fatigue, labor and garrison duty helped win over white soldiers to the arming of blacks. But it also placed a stigma of inferiority on black regiments. The stereotypes of the shuffling, banjo-strumming, happy-go-lucky darky caused many Northerners to doubt the...potential of blacks. Even some abolitionists wondered whether slaves who have been conditioned all their lives to fear and obey whites would stand in battle against those same whites.*[121]

McPherson goes on to discuss not only the stigma, but also the physical toll:

> *Although blacks fought in several major actions…they continued to do more garrison and fatigue duty and less fighting than white troops. This was reflected in the casualty rates of the two groups. Nearly 6 percent of white Union troops were killed in action, compared with 1.5 percent for black soldiers. On the other hand, the rate of death from disease among black troops (18 percent) was almost twice as high as among Northern white soldiers. As garrison troops, many black regiments had no chance for combat but suffered from the high disease rates typical of soldiers confined to one place, where their water supply turned foul and they built up deadly accumulations*

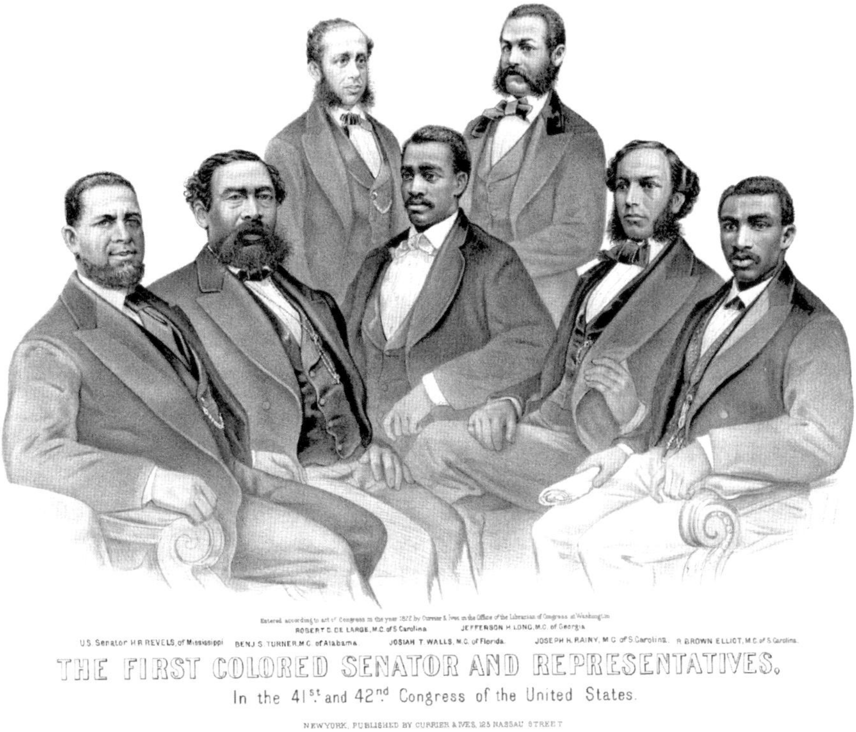

African American officer holders during Reconstruction. *Courtesy of the Library of Congress, Washington, D.C.*

> *of bacteria. Black regiments also received poorer medical care than whites. There were few black surgeons to draw upon…and white doctors were not notably eager to volunteer for black units.*[122]

During the war, the Union created a system for tracking soldiers. Each soldier had a card that recorded not only his location throughout the war, but also hospitalizations, location of hospitalizations, illnesses and other infirmities. Union clerks kept the cards current. This information was helpful on an individual level but also in the aggregate in order to tabulate information about all soldiers, both white and African American, during the wartime efforts. Unfortunately, the system broke down to a certain extent when soldiers were missing, taken as prisoners of war, killed in battle to the point of being unrecognizable or simply never located. Deserters were also a problem for the army in terms of numbers and calculating information. All of the factors make calculating accurate numbers difficult. Still, scholars have utilized the data to make helpful inferences. For example, historian Margaret Humphreys used supply levels as a gauge for casualties once a soldier died.[123]

Not surprisingly, the statistical picture with regard to African American casualties in the Union army is even less satisfactory than that for the organization as a whole. The reasons for this are many. The death reports were one major problem. It was routine for African American units not to report deaths but rather to enlist other soldiers, give them the names of the deceased and continue on as though the original soldier had never died. This is understandable because African Americans routinely came into the war lacking documentation about themselves. The lack of official record keeping made it possible for regiments to collect the undisbursed backpay of the deceased. It is important to note that, given the variety of sources for information regarding African American soldiers, there may be differences in terms of numbers, data and information.

Historian Herbert Aptheker has taken an exhaustive look at comparison numbers for African American and white troops. According to his calculations, the final Civil War report of the provost marshal general pointed out that the total loss was 314.65 casualties per 1,000.00 men for white volunteer troops. This number includes deaths, desertions and all types of discharges. The figure for African American troops was 290.82.[124]

If, however, an accounting is done for those killed in action plus those who died of disease only, the ratio for white volunteers is 94.32 per 1,000 soldiers and for African American troops 157.50 per 1,000. In terms of numbers, there were 2 million volunteer troops in the United States, with over 316,000 dying from the combined causes. The mortality rate for the white troops was 8.6 percent and for the African American troops was 20.5 percent.[125]

The greatest single cause of death for all troops was disease, and this was particularly true among the African American soldiers. The ratio of deaths from disease per 1,000 among the African American troops was over 140 while for the volunteer troops it was under 60. According to the surgeon general of the army, in his report of October 20, 1866, among white troops "the proportion of deaths, from all causes, to cases treated was one to every fifty-two," but with the African American troops "the mortality rate [was] one death to every twenty-nine cases treated."[126] Of the over two thousand regiments that made up the Union army—of which approximately 8 percent were African American—the Fifth United States Colored Heavy Artillery had the greatest number of injuries and death, with a total of 829 deaths. Of these, 124 occurred during battle, and 697 were due to disease and accidents.[127]

Early reports of Confederate prisons during the war were fairly positive. Where things began to go downhill was with the suspension of prisoners

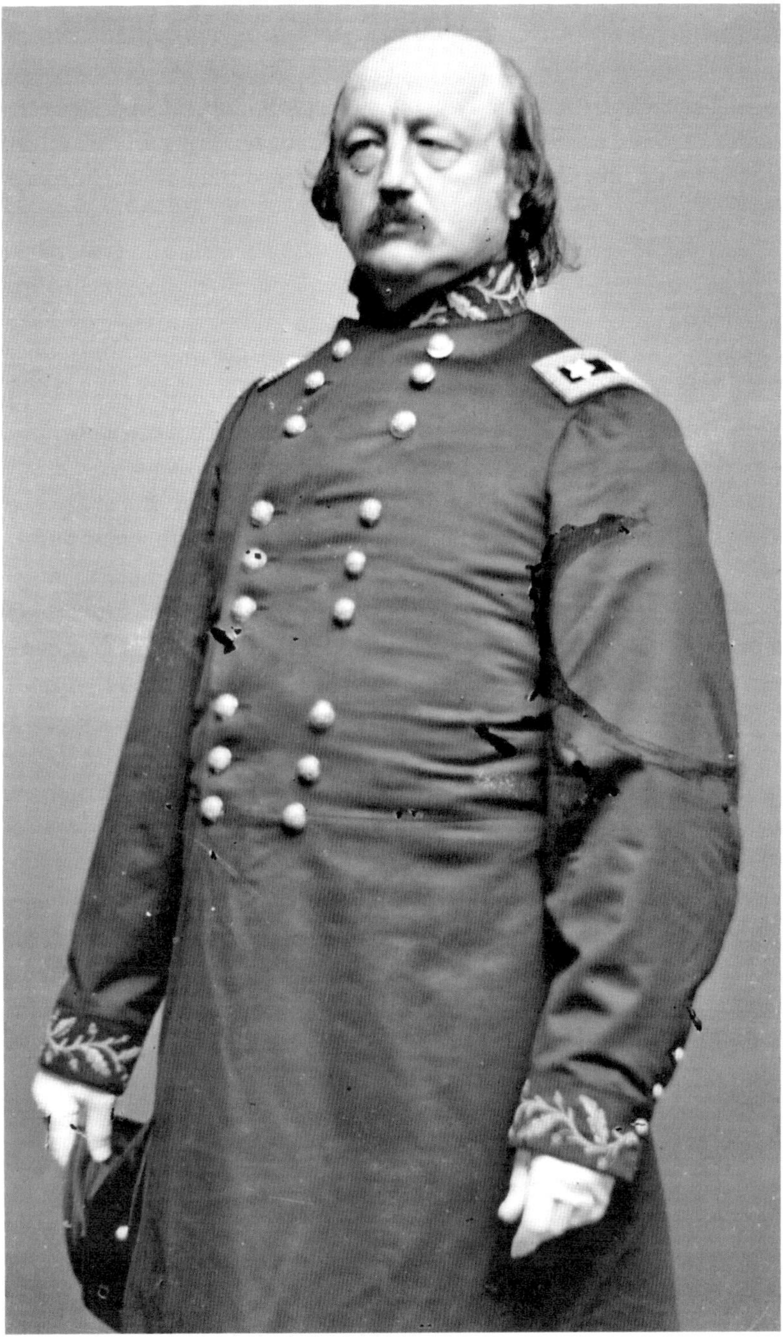

Major General Benjamin Franklin Butler. *Courtesy of the Library of Congress, Washington, D.C.*

in the summer of 1863. This caused overcrowding both in the prisons and prison hospitals. According to historian H.H. Cunningham, "An inspection of Belle Isle Prison Hospital in November, 1863, revealed that while the Federal patient received as much food, medicine and attention as the Confederate soldier in hospital he had only half as much room."[128] This was the same for prisons in Richmond and elsewhere.

Because of orders issued by Lieutenant General Ulysses S. Grant, there was no chance of release for exchange of prisoners until 1865. Meanwhile, the prisoners were placed on work details with duties such as the burial of men who died in the prison. William Marvel, in his study of Andersonville, acknowledges that some blacks received punishment by whipping but concluded, "The individual guards committed some petty cruelties against them but for the most part the prison authorities treated their black prisoners little differently than they did the white ones; they seemed to reserve their greatest animosity for the white officers who served with the Colored Troops."[129]

In 1862, General Benjamin Butler made a bold move with respect to his stance on slaves. Knowing that a South free of slaves would leave the Southern economy in utter ruin, he declared any slaves who were able to cross his lines to be contraband of war, appropriated in the same way as any other property of the enemy. Butler's policy was endorsed by the Union army. As word spread regarding such policies, and as troops moved through the South during 1862, droves of African Americans escaped behind the Union lines, with a growing number of individuals in camps with very few provisions. In the beginning of the war, slaves routinely made their way to D.C. African American women were utilized as cooks and nurses, among other duties. One use for African American men became manual labor necessary in an army camp. While many white officers believed that the utility of African American soldiers was in their ability to do fatigue duty and manual labor, that these men could also be of use with respect to actually fighting in the war was not lost on others in the army, especially given the investment that African Americans had in the outcome of the war.

In 1862, several commanders, from Major General David Hunter to Brigadier General Jim Lane, began to organize groups of ex-slaves for the purpose of serving in the army. There were also pockets of free African Americans who began to organize themselves to fight for their country.[130] While some of the military embraced the notion of African Americans taking up arms, others certainly did not. Samuel Kirkwood, governor of Iowa, stated to General Henry Halleck in August 1862 his own displeasure at the thought of African Americans fighting.[131] According to Humphreys, "Kirkwood may well have been responding to a law passed by Congress three weeks earlier. The law authorized the President to receive into the service of the United States, for the purpose of constructing entrenchments, or performing camp service, or any other labor or any military or naval service for which they may be found competent, persons of African descent, and such persons shall be enrolled and organized under such regulations...as the President may prescribe. This convoluted language emphasized the black man's role as a laborer but allowed for his induction as a regular soldier. The law further provided that if he was a slave to a person in rebellion, then he and his family shall forever after be free."[132]

Many African American recruits were ex-slaves straight from the plantation. The Union army compensated owners for removing African American males from the plantations. Additionally, the African American women who were left behind were required to do the work that their men would have done had they still been on the plantation. Plantation owners visited punishment and other forms of torture on the slave women when their male counterparts left for war. Slavery slowly died in the South over these years. The society built on the unpaid, punishing labor of African American men and women was ending.

Of some consequence in any consideration of African American casualties during the Civil War, was the policy adopted by the Confederate government in regard to African American troops. The Confederate government, until the end of 1864, did not consider African Americans as soldiers and, therefore, refused to treat them when captured in a manner similar to how other troops were treated. Confederate law required that African American prisoners be turned over to the authorities of the states from which they had been captured for trial by insurrectionists. White officers of African American units were subject to trial by court-martial, with death as a prescribed penalty. According to James Seddon, the Confederate secretary of war, he advised Lieutenant General E. Kirby Smith that white officers of African American soldiers, on capture, "had best be dealt with red-handed in the field or immediately thereafter." The official casualty figures report four officers of African regiments as having been "killed after capture," and another as having been "executed by the enemy."[133]

It appears that very few African Americans who had been free prior to enlistment were sold into slavery by the Confederacy, but they seem to have been confined, although not as confined as though they were prisoners of war.[134] It was, however, common procedure for the Confederacy to sell into slavery African Americans captured by its armies and declared to have been slaves prior to enlisting in the army. Where the masters were not found or did not appear, the armies utilized the African Americans as laborers.[135] African American soldiers had good reason to be concerned once captured by Confederate troops. Their fate, once in the hands of the Confederacy, was questionable at best and deadly at worst.[136]

This policy of refusing to view captured African Americans as soldiers for prisoner of war purposes was extremely problematic for the Union army. Furthermore, as stated elsewhere, it filled African American soldiers with a sense of the unknown that made engaging in battle that much more difficult.

As General Ullman remarked of his African American troops, "They are far more in earnest than we. I have talked with hundreds of them. They understand their position full as well as we do. They know the deep stake they have in the issue—that, if we are unsuccessful, they will be remanded to worse a slavery than before. They also have a settled conviction that if they are taken, they will be tortured and hung [*sic*]. These impressions will make them daring and desperate fighters."[137] Interestingly, it seems that because, once captured, African Americans' fates at the hands of the Confederates was such an unknown quantity, it made them fight that much harder. This added an additional level of stress for soldiers. Some of them found relief from such stressors through outlets such as alcohol.

Excessive drinking on the part of service members was a problem during the war. Mental and physical pain, loneliness, socializing with comrades and passing the time all contributed to drinking in most army camps.

Officers had various ways of dealing with the issue of alcohol in the camps. Some of the officers banned alcohol to thwart any drinking. From confiscating liquor in camps to donating alcohol to hospitals, officers were not above extreme means in order to stop the tide of drinking and alcohol consumption in their camps. Some abolitionists also blamed slave masters for using alcohol as a mechanism of control over their slaves, thus, leading to the problem that some African American soldiers had with alcohol consumption.[138]

From vows of abstinence to the formation of temperance organizations, regiments tried all manner of solutions to deal with the issue of soldiers and the alcohol problems.[139]

In Washington, D.C., confiscated alcohol was redistilled for use in shipping specimens to the Army Medical Museum.[140]

Authorities fashioned several ways to deal with soldiers who were excessively intoxicated. While being inebriated itself was not a crime, the ramifications of drunkenness potentially were. Punishment could be as severe as court-martial. The vast majority of soldiers were drunk occasionally; however, alcohol abuse was an issue in the Union army and also among the USCT officer corps.

Officers appear to have consumed more alcohol during the war than enlisted men, with officers seeming to believe that drinking was a "normal pastime."[141]

While soldiers chose to drink mainly whiskey, they would often drink whatever was available. At times, soldiers would receive whiskey in their ration as praise for a job well done or in order to keep them warm.[142]

When soldiers found it hard to obtain liquor in the camps, they would find other ways to get alcohol. From going to the nearest town to getting passes (ostensibly) to get supplies, soldiers who needed liquor would find local bars or other venues from which to get it. If desperate enough, soldiers would steal alcohol from local townspeople. Some local townspeople would sneak liquor to troops directly. This would often lead to the soldiers becoming unruly and being confined in the guardhouse. According to author Schroeder-Lein, "Foraging for supplies in enemy country means raiding stashed liquor, as well as food. Temptation was often closer to home. Alcoholic beverages were believed to have medicinal value as tonics and stimulants for the sick and wounded. Alcohol also served as a base to which various powdered medications such as quinine, were added."[143]

Regimental doctors and other healthcare workers were not immune to raids by soldiers in desperate need of an alcoholic drink. Hospitals, both field and general, had supplies of alcohol such as whiskey. Doctors had canteens of whiskey to take into the field to tend to the wounded soldiers in desperate need of relief; such supplies would occasionally be stolen and used by regimental soldiers for nonmedicinal purposes. "Getting barrels of alcohol from the medical source to the field or hospital was quite problematic, especially when soldiers knew the contents of the barrel and had no compunction about emptying the barrels and replacing the contents with water.[144]

Some surgeons became crafty in order to combat pilfering of their alcohol supply. When Union assistant surgeon John H. Brinton noticed that the barrels of alcohol that he sent to the front lines for preserving specimens of wounds for the Army Medical Museum were being taken, he decided to put tartar emetic in the alcohol, thus causing sickness and vomiting in anyone who ingested it. Brinton had no further problems with his supply.[145]

Unfortunately, it was not only the soldiers who were prone to taking alcohol inappropriately. In the hospitals, alcohol had a way of disappearing due in large measure to attendants, from nurses to surgeons to laundresses. Whether alcohol was stolen for personal use or in order to be sold to a desperate soldier at some later point, keeping order over alcohol in the hospital was difficult if not impossible. Drunkenness in the hospital setting on the part of the healthcare workers was not unusual.

What were the ramifications for individuals who either stole alcohol or used it to excess? There were a variety of punishments. As stated earlier, some alcohol that was confiscated was used for shipping specimens, a vital service, especially for surgeons at the front. If a soldier was drunk, he might find his punishment that of spending a night in the guardhouse. An officer with serious, lasting alcohol problems might actually face court-martial. The medical director of General Hospitals for the Confederate Army of Tennessee, Samuel H. Stout, gave soldiers who were found to be inebriated two choices: resigning commission or court-martial. Although there are no exact figures, alcohol abuse created many problems for both the Union and Confederate armies. From May 1861 to June 1865, 124 white Union soldiers were discharged from the army by surgeons who deemed them disabled from alcohol abuse. Almost twenty Federal generals were relieved of their duties because of alcohol-related problems.[146]

Moving from alcohol problems to overall disease rates, soldiers of the USCT suffered from disease at different and higher rates than their white counterparts. Some of this, as the wonderful historian Andrew Black demonstrates, can be attributed to issues of environment and location as well as the kind of duty that they were forced to endure. Additional factors include, as have already been alluded to, medical experiences during slave time and the type of treatment that African American soldiers received from Union physicians and other healthcare workers.[147]

The numbers, as we have seen, vary with respect to numbers of fatalities, wounds and disease during the war. Historian Andrew Black's numbers state that fatalities from all causes during the war exceeded 300,000 men. The numbers for white troops were 90,638 killed in battle or because of wounds and 171,806 from disease. For African American troops, 3,331 died in battle or because of wounds and 29,963 from disease. It is interesting to note that because of the level of sickness among the troops, it would seem that the "normal" state for both many white troops and African American troops was one of being ill.[148]

While there were geographical differences throughout the war with respect to the frequency and virulence of various diseases, the fact is that both white and African American soldiers died in disproportionate numbers from disease as opposed to wounds or injuries. The biggest culprit of death in camps was diarrhea and dysentery, also known as "camp fever."

Dysentery is rarely seen in developed countries and has its roots more squarely located in third-world countries. It is an intestinal disease mainly of the colon that causes a chemical irritant, bacteria, protozoa or parasites in the victim. Where there is a lack of clean, safe water and food, diseases such as this can develop. There are various forms that the disease can take, being classified as acute diarrhea, chronic diarrhea, acute dysentery and chronic dysentery.[149] These four diseases alone accounted for more illness and death in camps than any others. They were prevalent at the beginning of the war and stayed until the end and beyond.

These diseases were very prevalent in Andersonville and other prisons. Upward of 25 percent of African Americans who died from a disease died from one of these four diseases, and it is unclear whether all of these diseases were separate diseases as opposed to one horrible disease with various stages, all of which the victims suffered until death. According to Black, "Out of black mortality of 29,963, due to disease, those reported in this classification amounted to 6,764 or 22.57 percent of the total. Of these, 1,368 were attributed to acute diarrhea, 3,278 to chronic diarrhea, 1,492 to acute dysentery and 626 to chronic dysentery."[150] Furthermore, the suffering that accompanied these diseases did not end with the cessation of wartime efforts. Ex-soldiers would go on to suffer from a dysentery-like disease long after the war was over, and innumerable deaths accompanied such suffering. According to Black, "Dysentery, the class of disease with the highest rate of mortality for both white and black troops, did not originate with the idiosyncrasies of any one group of troops. Instead, it derived from the level of social development and patterns of settlement of all soldiers which were as easily associated with white troops as black, thereby explaining the lack of difference in the rates of suffering."[151]

Other profound killers of African American and white soldiers alike were pneumonia and typhoid. The numbers and severity for pneumonia-like diseases in African Americans were more virulent than in white soldiers, but the diseases were extremely deadly in both populations, meaning 20.69 percent of total deaths were attributable to respiratory diseases. With respect to white troops, the numbers were 17,896 deaths or 10.42 percent.[152] Caretakers of the soldiers were not immune from such diseases. Author Louisa May Alcott—who served as a nurse in Washington, D.C., during the war—contracted typhoid fever during the war, was treated with mercury and suffered the side effects of the disease and treatment her entire life.[153]

With respect to white troops, after diarrhea and dysentery, typhoid and malaria were the largest killers. They were often interlinked because of the difficulty that physicians had in separating out the two diseases, with typhoid and malaria often being mistaken for each other. Some physicians believed that the two diseases were interlinked and possibly caused each other. Typhoid and malaria were described as "typho-malarial fever," "typhoid fever," "typhus fever" and other diseases that would appear to fall somewhere on the malaria continuum.[154] The thought at the time was that these diseases were caused by foul or polluted air, leading again to assumptions about means of contraction that were flawed at best and inaccurate at worst.[155]

Adding to the difficulty was the symptomatology of diseases. Several of these diseases were distinct in their disease process. Fevers were of various duration, levels of seriousness and temperature. Some individuals had fevers lasting several days, others longer, with the fevers being of varying quality, which often went unnoticed by physicians during that time. This only added to the problem of distinguishing various diseases based on symptomatology.[156]

The next class of diseases, in terms of mortality, is known as eruptive fevers. This class includes measles, smallpox and scarlet fever. Smallpox was the largest killer in this group, with 2,341,000 deaths attributable to this disease. Overall, deaths from such diseases accounted for 3,521 deaths, 11.75 percent of disease mortality. It is interesting to note that the eruptive fevers are childhood diseases, but soldiers from rural areas that had not previously been exposed to such diseases or from areas where the diseases did not occur were susceptible as adults. Depending on where an individual soldier came from—a rural setting or a city—would indicate the likelihood of his being struck down by this class of diseases. Whole regiments could be infected in such a manner.[157] Although smallpox was able to be prevented through individuals' being vaccinated, many soldiers were not protected against the disease when the Civil War began.[158]

From an epidemiological standpoint, it is instructive to recognize and examine the causes that led to African Americans and whites suffering from different diseases at varying rates and varying levels of seriousness. Because there was a limited understanding of germs and microbes, physicians were strained in terms of understanding and ascertaining the root cause of diseases in general and why such diseases were more prevalent in certain groups and less so in others. Given the stresses of war, it was all but impossible to do an in-depth prevalence study on the soldiers during the war. Practitioners understood that there was something important about cleanliness in camps and these led to better health outcomes than soldiers living in filth, but the precise mechanisms of this were less well understood.[159]

The other factor leading to disease transmission was the soldiers' level of understanding about public health and medicine. With the number of under-educated young boys fighting—and with habits of childhood difficult to break, especially with no clear reason to—the ability to bring change was close to impossible.

Why did African American troops suffer from pneumonia at rates so much higher than white troops? It is instructive to go back to the disease status of African American troops when they entered the war. Many African Americans, being just barely out of slavery, had suffered mightily from disease and public health issues in ways very different from those of their white counterparts. Beyond the obvious diet and nutrition issues, there were also the issues of overcrowding among the slaves and interaction with others. In the South, whites had a limited sphere of individuals with whom they came into contact. For African Americans, the situation was quite different. In addition to all the whites they encountered, they also lived in extremely tight, overcrowded situations. Even the poorest whites in the South had quarters more spacious than those of their African American counterparts.[160]

The crowded slave quarters were a perfect breeding ground for respiratory diseases such as pneumonia. Interestingly, it would be this same type of confinement that African Americans and whites alike would find themselves in during the war. Given the exposure that many African Americans had prior to the war, their rate of reinfection was extremely high—many whites had not experienced these respiratory diseases.

Paradoxically, there was a notion among white soldiers that African Americans had the ability to somehow overcome disease, hard work, fatigue duty and other stressors at a much higher rate than their white counterparts. Due to the level and severity of labor that African American soldiers participated in during the war, the healthcare outcomes were much poorer. Worse health on entering the war, coupled with hard labor during the war and lack of sufficient healthcare, led to a trifecta conflagration of circumstances for these troops that was not conducive to good health.[161]

Adjutant General Lorenzo Thomas was ordered by President Lincoln to raise troops from the large groups of ex-slaves who followed the Union army. On one such trip, he reported to Secretary of War Stanton that he had succeeded in recruiting 56,320 men. In the same report, he discusses the part that African American soldiers were expected to fill—namely, that of laborers—and how this would impact their overall health.

According to Black:

> *Where white and black troops come together in the same command the later* [sic] *have to do the work. At first this was always the case, and in vain did I endeavor to correct it, contending that if they were to be made soldiers, time would have to be afforded for drill and discipline, and that they should have only their fair share of fatigue duty. The prejudice in the army against their employment as troops was very great; but now, since the blacks have fully shown their fighting qualities and manliness it has greatly changed.*[162]

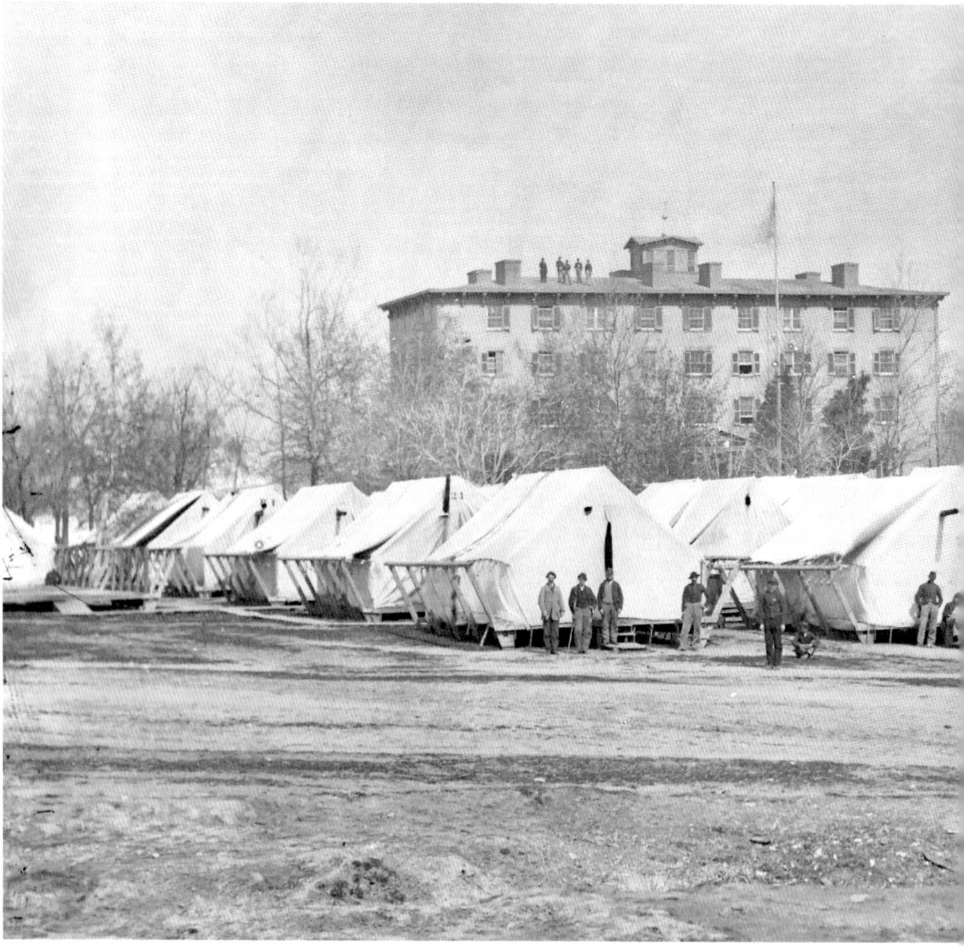

Hospital tents in the rear of Douglas Hospital in Washington, D.C. *Courtesy of the Library of Congress, Washington, D.C.*

As the war continued, the overall health outcomes of African American troops actually improved. This can be attributed to several factors, with two of the most important being the lessening of arduous fatigue duty and better overall care by physicians assigned to USCT regiments.[163] Thomas Wentworth Higginson, commander of a USCT regiment, stated:

> *In what respect were the colored troops a source of disappointment?...In one respect only, that of health. Their health improved, indeed, as they grew more familiar with military life; but I think that neither their physical nor*

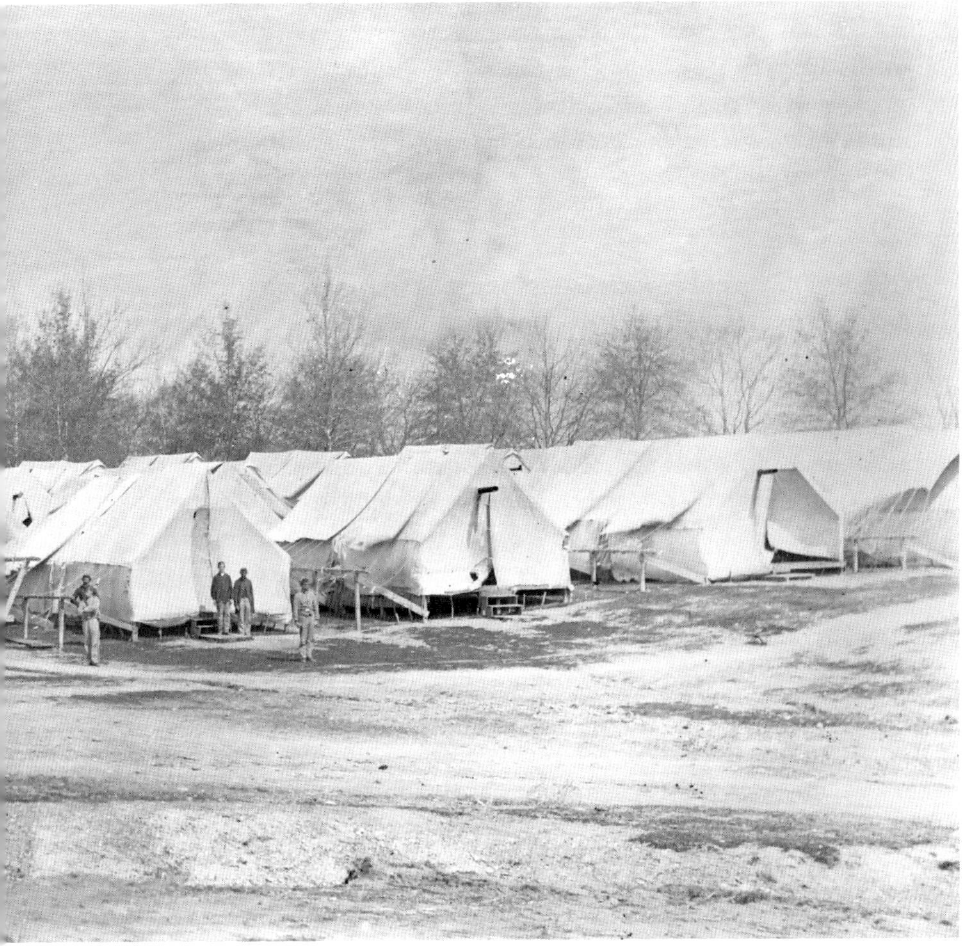

moral temperament gave them that toughness, that obstinate purpose of living, which sustains the more materialistic [white soldier]. *They had not, to be sure, the same predominant diseases, suffering in the pulmonary, not in the digestive organs; but they suffered a good deal. They felt malaria less, but they were more easily choked by dust and made ill by dampness. On the other hand they submitted more readily to sanitary measures than whites, and with efficient officers, were more easily kept clean. They were injured throughout the army by an undue share of fatigue duty, which is*

> *not only exhausting but demoralizing to a soldier; by the unsuitableness of the rations, which gave them salt meat instead of rice and hominy; and by the lack of good medical attendance. Their childlike constitutions needed prompt and efficient surgical care; but almost all the colored troops were enlisted late in the war, when it was hard to get good surgeons for any regiments, and especially for these.*[164]

The regiment having the second-greatest number of deaths in the entire army was the Sixty-fifth United States Colored Infantry. Interestingly, this regiment did not participate in active engagement. The deaths in this regiment were from disease and accidents. Of a total of 755 persons, 6 were officers.[165] The regiment with the fourth-highest number of deaths was the Fifty-sixth United States Colored Infantry, with a total of 25 killed in battle and 649 dying of disease. There were 6 officers among the dead for this regiment.[166]

A critical examination of the state of the health of African American soldiers during the war would be remiss without looking at the heavy death rates among the regiments and the explanation for these rates. According to the army's provost marshal general, in offering reasons for the lower death rate from disease among officers than among enlisted men, many of the distinctions he makes in the conditions confronting enlisted men as compared to commissioned officers applied to African Americans and whites.

> *Officers are better sheltered than men; and their food is generally better in quality and more varied in kind. They are not so much crowded to gather in tents and quarters. They have superior advantages in regard to personal cleanliness. As prisoners of war, too, they were generally treated more leniently. Another favoring circumstance, and by no means the least potential, was the superior morale.*[167]

Lorenzo Thomas, when writing to Secretary Stanton in Washington, D.C., to report on his recruiting trips, spoke about the hardships in recruiting medical officers for African American regiments. Because of a lack of actual physicians, this left regiments in a situation where assistants and others took the place of surgeons for purposes of administering care to these regiments.[168]

Malaria was a disease experienced differently by African Americans than by whites and took its toll on Washington, D.C. Historian Andrew K. Black points to Peter Wood's discussion of the disease and the influence of sickle-

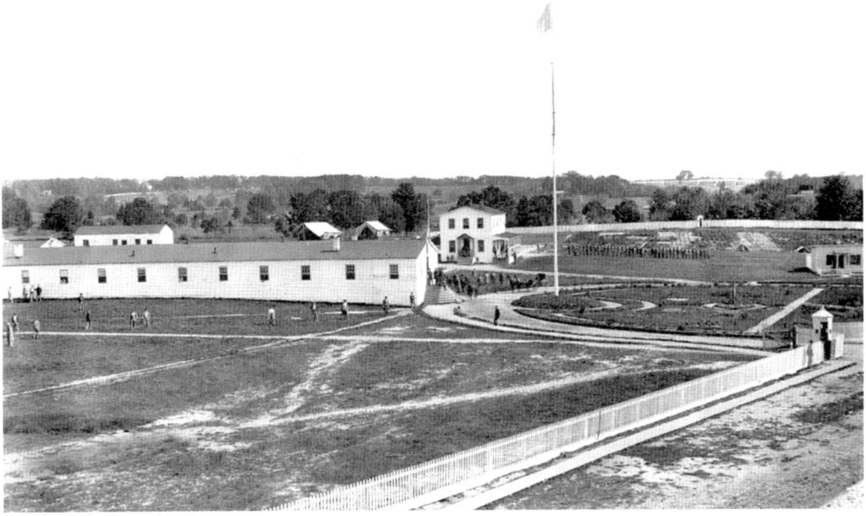

Campbell Hospital in Washington, D.C., in the 1860s. *Courtesy of the Historical Society of Washington, D.C.*

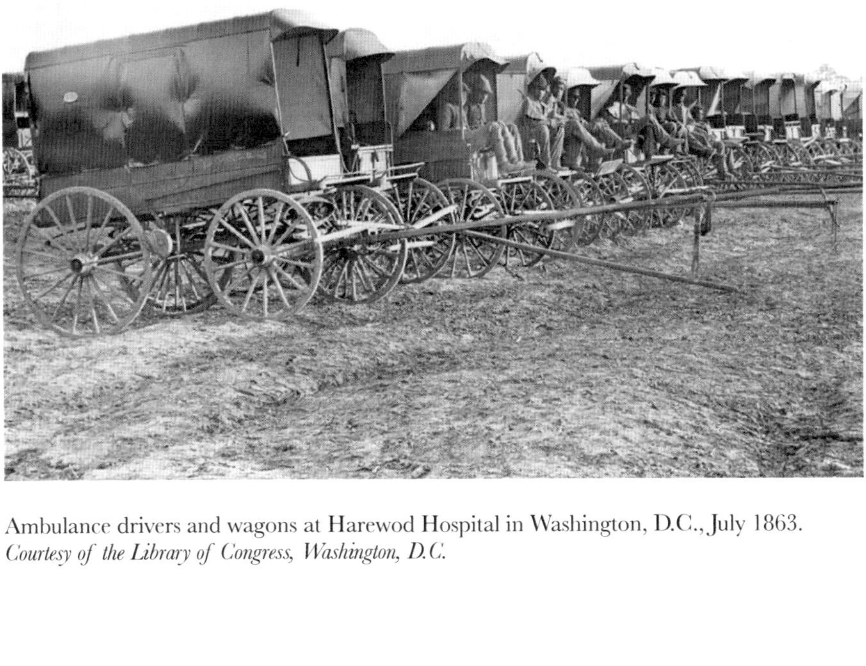

Ambulance drivers and wagons at Harewod Hospital in Washington, D.C., July 1863. *Courtesy of the Library of Congress, Washington, D.C.*

cell anemia as the deciding factor in the differences that African Americans and whites experienced. This theory seems ripe for reexamination. The sickle-cell carrier trait that Wood credits for this difference does indeed provide greater protection for a carrier than for a noncarrier. However, only a portion of the African American population were actually carriers, while 100 percent had been exposed to malaria in their environment.

Traditionally, malaria had been endemic throughout North America from the time of the European conquest. By 1850, however, it had been eradicated in New England. Since mosquitos, the mechanisms for transmission for malaria, died out in the frost each year, only a new source of infection in the spring made possible a continuance of the endemic presence. The Northern Mississippi Valley retained an endemic presence as a result of its trade with the areas bordering the southern part of the river. In contrast, as trade with the Caribbean began to be centered in New Orleans rather than New York, Philadelphia or Boston and the sources of renewed springtime infection left with the changing patterns of trade, malaria disappeared from all but isolated pockets of New England. At the same time, no annual frost killed mosquitos in the South, and the infection remained as an endemic presence throughout the region. Black goes on to state:

> *Consequently, blacks generally came from the part of the country where they had an almost one hundred percent likelihood to have been exposed to malaria and acquired some resistance. Since white troops mostly came from regions where it was either unusual, or where the type of malaria was different from that in the South, they faced the southern disease environment with little or no resistance. Since the greatest resistance to malaria for an entire population comes from acquired immunity, Wood's theory that a genetic factor only present in a portion of the black population was responsible for their greater resistance entirely ignores epidemiologically important geographical and environmental factors.*[169]

Neither side had an organized system of removing the wounded from the field when the Civil War began. Although some ambulances were available through the army's quartermaster department, those accompanying the Union forces to the first Battle of Bull Run, for example, on July 21, 1861, were driven by civilians, many of whom either left their posts or were intoxicated, thus being unable to take the wounded back to Washington, D.C. These soldiers had to be transported on a wagon train back to Washington, D.C., several days later. The suggestion of an ambulance corps was put forth, but there was no movement on this front. Due in large measure to these uncoordinated efforts, Union troops suffered greatly because of badly coordinated evacuations of the sick and wounded. A wounded soldier was more likely to receive treatment in time if some of his comrades took him to a medical station or field hospital. This was, of course, very inefficient because while the wounded man was carried out of harm's way to receive medical attention, several other soldiers were out of commission while bringing the wounded man to safety and help. This is true of Washington, D.C., as soldiers were often brought to D.C. directly for care from other battlefields.

It would not be until the summer of 1862 that an ambulance corps was finally established. Each ambulance was supposed to have a driver and two stretcher bearers with the rank of private. First lieutenants directed the ambulances, and sergeants were in charge of the regimental ambulances with the ambulance service designed to be headed by a captain. Each regiment was assigned one medical supply transportation cart, one four-horse ambulance and two two-horse ambulances. The ambulances of each division would stay together to be used solely for medical purposes, under the control of the medical director. Having such rules in place would stop the problem of quartermasters commandeering ambulances for nonmedical uses, such as hauling officers' baggage. One of the most important aspects of having an ambulance corps was that unwounded soldiers would no longer be responsible for caring for their fallen comrades and making sure they were removed from the battlefield. There would now be trained individuals in place to ensure that the wounded received the kind of care and assistance they needed.[170]

The Battle of Antietam on September 17, 1862, was the first testing ground for the new ambulance system to see how effective it would prove to be in battle. With a corps that was still a work in progress, three hundred ambulances managed to clear the wounded from the field in two days. In the Battle of Fredericksburg in December 1862, nearly one thousand ambulances removed the wounded from the field in twelve hours. The question arose as to whether ambulances would be effective in western armies. While Surgeon General William A. Hammond recommended that an ambulance corps should be established for such armies, both Secretary of War Edwin Stanton and Union army commander Henry W. Halleck rejected the notion. Regardless, on March 30, 1863, General Ulysses S. Grant issued General Orders No. 22, setting up an ambulance corps for the Army of the Tennessee. On March 11, 1864, the United States Congress passed legislation making the ambulance corps official. Soon after, General Orders No. 106 was

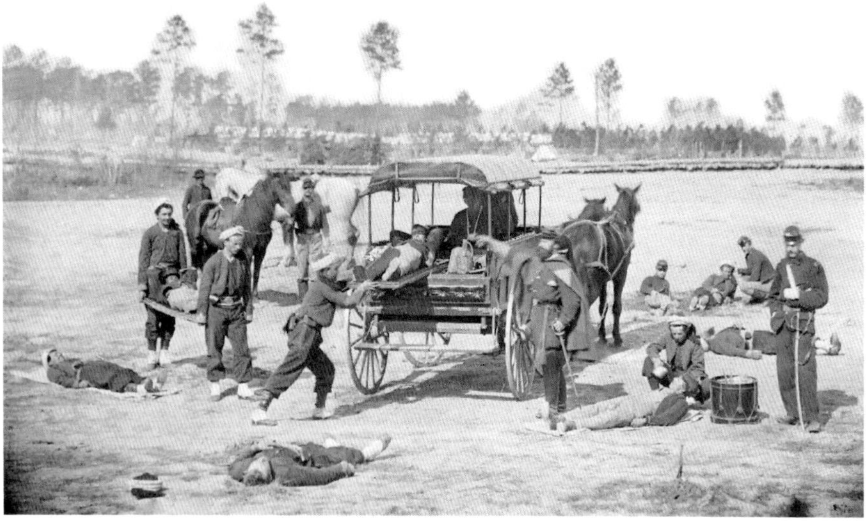

A Civil War ambulance removing the wounded. *Courtesy of the Library of Congress, Washington, D.C.*

issued, which solidified the army ambulance corps. The armies were already ahead of the politicians, and as of April 1864, the ambulance corps of the Union army's Fifth Corps consisted of 17 commissioned officers, 550 enlisted men, 171 two-horse ambulances, 62 supply wagons, 11 medicine wagons 528 horses and 348 mules.[171]

It is clear that, as a rule, the weapons provided to African American troops were of a poor quality. Memoranda from the inspector general's department comment on the fact that, while African American units were usually equal to others in discipline and conduct, their actual efficiency was curtailed because the arms within several regiments were of different kinds.[172]

Brigadier General J. Hawkins, commanding the First Brigade, USCT, requested that the War Department issue appropriate weapons to the African American troops. The next month, the assistant secretary of war declared that the department had never intended "that the colored soldiers should be armed with inferior weapons." He asserted that his belief that the foreign arms turned in by another commander, repaired by ordinance and now in the hands of Hawkins's men could not "be properly called inferior," but he added that since "your officers and men think otherwise," new muskets would be forwarded "as soon as they can be."[173]

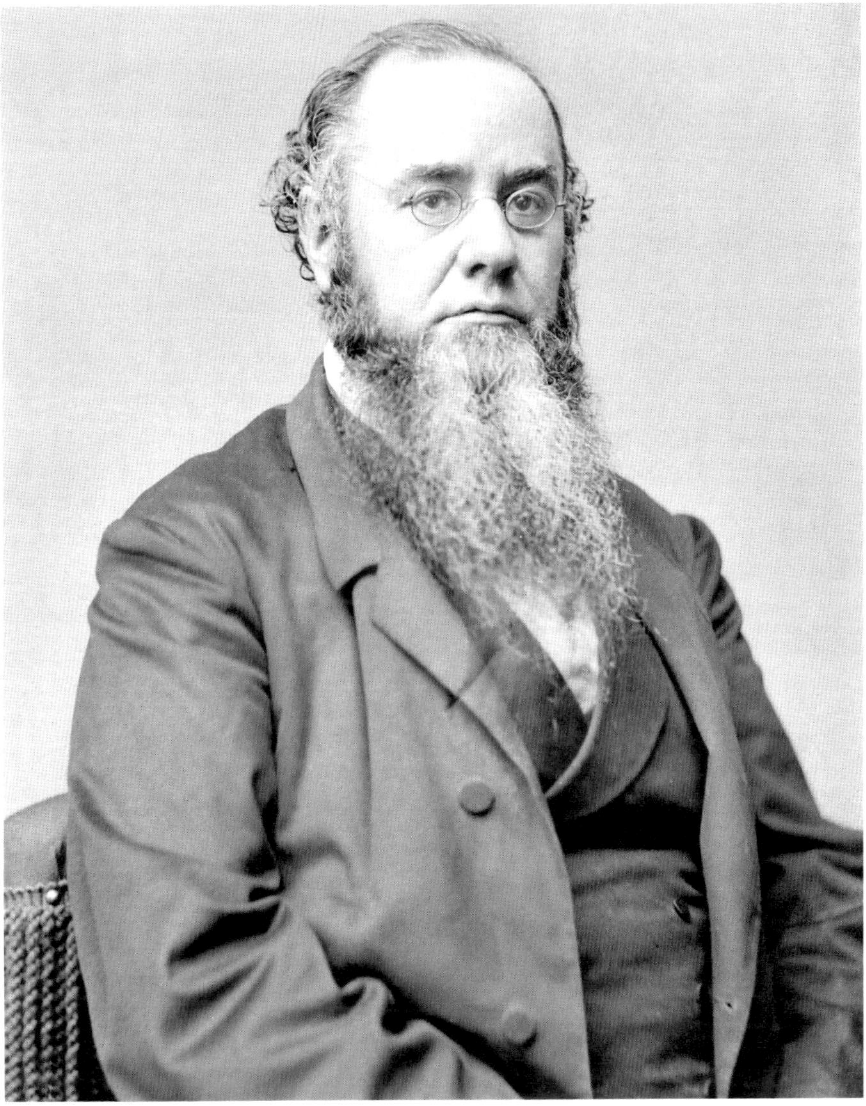

Edwin Stanton, secretary of war. *Courtesy of the Library of Congress, Washington, D.C.*

African American soldiers received inferior weaponry to their white counterparts because of the notion that regiments who were going to be engaged in more combat should have better arms than those regiments who were not as engaged in combat. This argument clearly had less and less merit as the war continued, and African American regiments

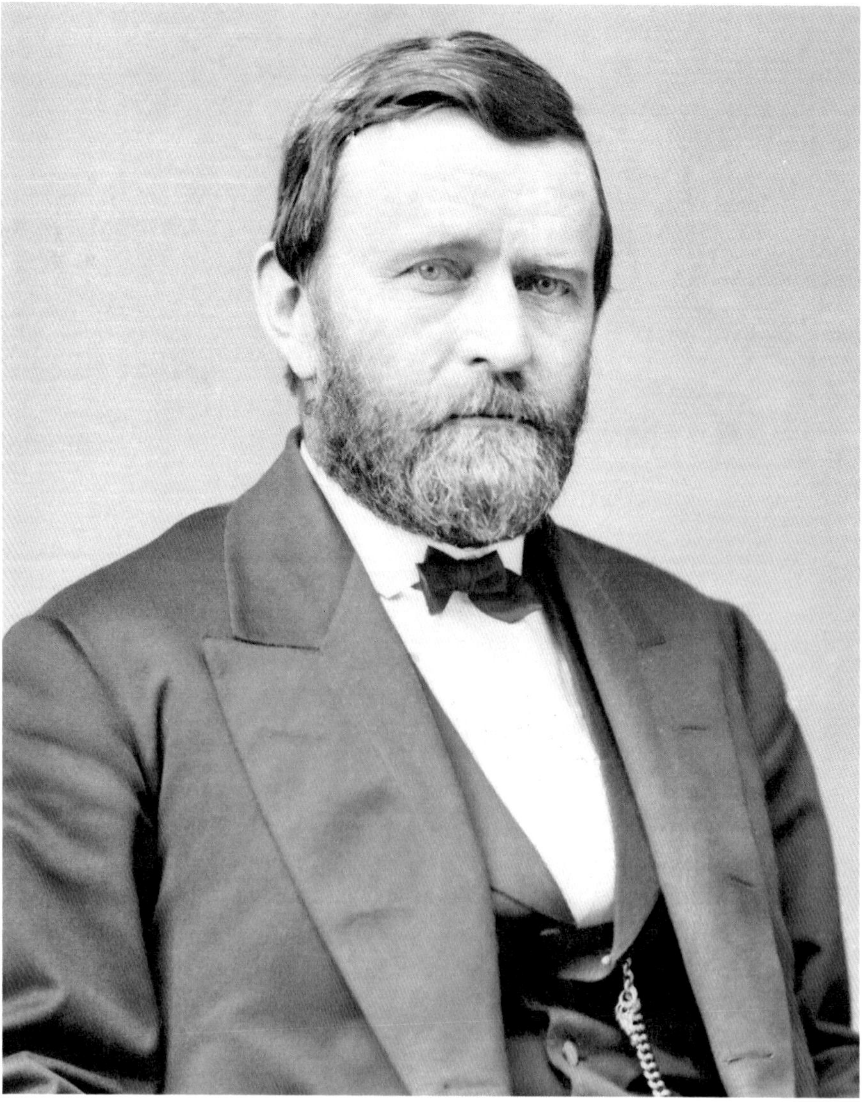

General Ulysses S. Grant. *Courtesy of the Library of Congress, Washington, D.C.*

demonstrated themselves repeatedly to be more than up to the task of active duty. According to Wilson, "It was argued that the best troops should have the best arms, and since white soldiers were considered superior to black soldiers the blacks were generally given inferior weaponry." He goes on to state that Major Edward Cameron expressed this view succinctly in an inspection report from August 1863. Commenting on General Edward Wild's African Brigade, Major Cameron declared, "Colored troops as far as I have seen are not equal to white ones…It is not intended I presume to put first class arms into their hands but I would recommend that some of the Austrian rifles now at the depot on Morris Island also be substituted for the unserviceable ones which they have now."[174]

Given the fact that many of the African American soldiers had little to no experience with taking up arms, the fact that they might be given inferior weapons was infuriating to the majority of their superior officers. Some commanding officers described in detail the issues with giving African American soldiers inferior weapons. First, most African Americans entering service had never held a weapon. Giving them deficient weapons would be of a greater disservice than doing so with a soldier who had weaponry experience and might be able to adjust to such problems because of experience with arms. This, of course, would lead to more casualties and injuries. Second, in order for soldiers to truly become better soldiers, they had to have the time to drill and practice with proper equipment. Doing so with subpar equipment was a waste of time at best and dangerous at worst.[175]

Some commanding officers pointed to inferior weaponry as the reason why battles and, more importantly, lives were lost. That these soldiers were fighting with such armaments meant that they were unable to properly engage in battle and also unable to properly defend themselves. If a unit was well armed, it benefited the entire unit, both African American soldiers and their white officers. In a letter from Brigadier General William Birney to Major C.W. Foster, he railed against the poor armaments of his soldiers, citing that such tactics on the part of the government did a disservice to his unit and the army as a whole. "All this is very stupid. Is the Government to keep whole regiments under pay with arms that won't go off? How was this any different than having soldiers murdered outright?" Birney queried. He pointed to a much more nefarious culprit at play: the bigotry of certain individuals in positions to make such decisions that overrode good sense and their duty to the Union.[176]

Due to several reports regarding infractions against African American troops, the adjutant general's office began an investigation into how African American troops were treated. It was brought to light that excessive fatigue details were still assigned African American troops but that it was not as egregious work as had been during earlier phases of the war; however, it was noted that African American troops were still used excessively for fatigue and labor details.[177]

William Cullen Bryant was so influenced by Brigadier General Ullman's charges of abuse towards his African American unit that he decided to place the matter, officially, before the army's adjutant general:

> *There is a topic* [he declared] *to which I desire to draw your attention. Doubtless you have already considered it. So far, colored troops in this Department* [of the Gulf], *have been used chiefly for fatigue duty. I much fear, unless there shall be a radical change, they never will be otherwise used in this Department. I have been striving for the year past to obtain an opportunity to bring my special command into shape as soldiers, not laborers. The 1st Brigade of my Division was ordered to the front some three weeks ago. I learn they are used simply on "fatigue duty." I humbly suggest, then, they should not be kept in the background, and continue to be kept degraded as simply laborers. If they are thus treated in the future, as they have been in the past, we may be sure their morale will be entirely destroyed.*[178]

The enforcement provision of this order declared: "Commanders of Colored Troops, in cases where the troops under their commands are required to perform an excess of labor above white troops in the same command, will represent the case to the common superior, through the regular channels."[179]

A brigadier general sent on an inspection tour of African American units reported in December 1863 that the quality of their officers, though lately improved, was still poor. Another general, himself commanding African American troops, declared in the same period, "I well know that those prophets who declare that negroes never will make soldiers are striving to force their prophecies to work out their own fulfillment, by appointing ignoramuses and boors to be officers over men who are as keen-sighted as any to notice the shortcomings of those placed over them. Men have been made Field Officers in this section, who are not fit to be non-commissioned officers."[180]

Another reference to the appointment of officers in African American units who were subpar occurs in a somewhat earlier letter to President Lincoln in D.C. from one Major A.E. Borey, the provost marshal of the Norfolk-Portsmouth area in Virginia. Major Borey assured the president that the

> *majority of our officers of all grades have no sympathy with your policy* [of enlisting African Americans and emancipating slaves]; *nor with*

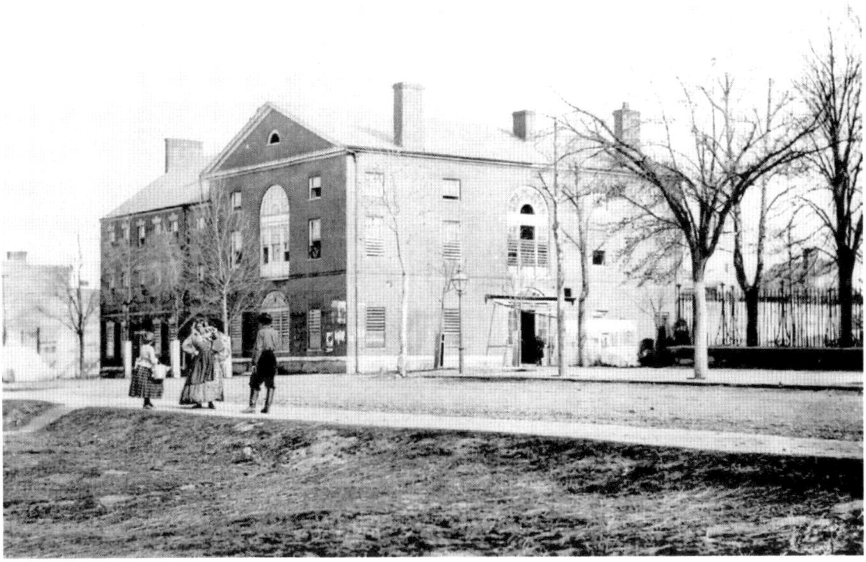

Old Capitol Prison, Washington, D.C. *Courtesy of the United States National Archives and Records Administration.*

> *anything human. They hate the African American more than they love the Union and you would probably suppose that such men would not seek or accept positions in the African American Regts.; not so however. There is a regular cabal here among the very worst class of African American hating officers, to secure & parcel out to themselves & others like themselves, all those places. These men have at this moment two agents in Washington under pay—sent there from here—to secure the appointments in this force, all the way down from Brigadier to Captain. For God's sake don't let this black Army fall into such hands.*[181]

Odd types of punishments also existed for soldiers, white and African American. Brutality—beating, bucking, gagging or hanging by thumbs—occasionally characterized the treatment of all soldiers, with African American soldiers receiving the brunt of the harshness. Pouring molasses over a man's body and having the soldier stay outside all day was not unheard of. This was something that mainly African American troops endured.[182]

In the spring of 1865, Laura Haviland, abolitionist and reformer, was named inspector of hospitals by General Oliver O. Howard, commissioner of the

Freedmen's Bureau. Her duties in Washington, D.C., included distribution of supplies, reporting on living conditions of those in the hospitals, volunteering as a nurse and advocating for the case of African Americans.[183] In her autobiography *A Woman's Life-works: Labors and Experiences of Laura S. Haviland*, Haviland speaks about her work in and around Washington, D.C., stating:

> *On September 20th, I visited a number of sick that I supplied with bedding and clothing. I walked six miles that day, and then went to the office of the Freedmen's Bureau, where I was furnished with an ambulance and driver to take things to the sufferers I had visited. After spending several days in this war, visiting schools and giving attention to many sufferers. I returned, weary in body but restful in mind, and thankful that the friends of humanity had made me the almoner of their gifts.*[184]

While many treated the wounded African American soldier with the greatest of care, the atrocities that some African American soldiers suffered cannot be ignored. Much of this inferior treatment was due in large part to the beliefs at the time regarding African Americans and their status in society. Even in the Union army, where white soldiers and healthcare workers were fighting for the rights of African Americans, African American soldiers who understood in their own way the connection between diet and health, indicated the army rations as one source of deteriorating health. When looking at poor health outcomes for African American soldiers, it's obvious that both the quality and quantity of the food they received are to blame. According to a private, African Americans routinely congregated "around our cookhouse to get what bean or pea soup we leave. It is allowed in plentiful quantities by government and goes begging with us, but they receive it with eagerness and swallow it with voracity. Bread is served them only once a week they tell me."[185]

In addition to all the other indignities that African American soldiers had to deal with—poor training, faulty equipment, lack of adequate leadership and lack of sufficient nutrients—once they actually saw fighting, there was a question as to whether that kind of fighting led to even more casualties than all the reasons described above. Even the Confederate soldiers noted that it appeared African American soldiers were used as the first attack in battles as the war went on, with reinforcements coming in the form of white troops.

The relationship between low morale and high casualties, particularly from disease, seems to be so close that it must be addressed and the overall issues of morale and disease examined. One cause of low morale was the discrimination practiced by the government against its African American soldiers in the matter of pay. As referenced in more detail on page forty-nine, all African American troops, regardless of rank, from 1862 to 1864 were offered a monthly wage of ten dollars minus three dollars for clothing, which was three dollars less than that paid white privates, who had no clothing costs. This was done even though African American recruits had been officially and repeatedly assured, on multiple occasions and by high military and civilian officials, that they would receive the same pay, equipment and rations as every other United States volunteer.[186]

Long after pay was retroactively reinstated for African American soldiers, these men continued to fight for equality. The pay that African American soldiers received had a direct effect on the war efforts and their health during the war.[187]

The refugee camps needed guards to keep intruders out and to police the activities of the refugees themselves. The Federal soldiers almost unanimously objected to performing such service. (They had enlisted to save the Union, not to guard a milling herd of bewildered African Americans.) It seemed logical, after a time, to raise guard detachments from among the African Americans themselves, outfitting them with castoff army uniforms. Then it appeared that the immense reserve of manpower represented by the newly freed slaves might be put to more direct use. At last the government authorized, and even encouraged, the organization of African American regiments, to be officered by whites but to be regarded as troops of the line, available for combat duty if needed. To this move the soldiers made a good deal of objections—at first. According to authors Richard Ketchum and Bruce Catton:

> *Then they began to change their minds. They did not like Negroes, for race prejudice of a malignity rarely seen today was very prevalent in the North at that time, and they did not want to associate with them on anything remotely like terms of equality, but they came to see that much might be said for Negro regiments. For one thing, a great many enlisted men in the Northern armies could win officers' commissions in these regiments, and a high private who saw a chance to become a lieutenant or a captain was likely to lose a great deal of his antagonism to the notion of Negro soldiers. More important than this was the dawning realization that the colored soldier could stop a Rebel bullet just as well as a white soldier could, and when he did so some white soldier who would otherwise have died would go on living…And so by the middle of 1863 the North was raising numbers of Negro regiments, and the white soldiers who had been so bitter about the*

> *idea adjusted themselves rapidly. All told, the federals put more than one hundred and fifty-thousand Negroes into uniform. Many of these regiments were used only for garrison duty, and in some other cases the army saw to it that the colored regiments became little more than permanent fatigue details to relieve white soldiers of hard work, but some units saw actual combat service and in a number of instances acquitted themselves well. And there was an importance to this that went far beyond any concrete achievements on the field of battle, for this was the seed of further change. The war had freed the slave, the war had put freed slaves into army uniform—and a permanent alteration in the colored mans' status would have to come out of that fact. Many who had worn the country's uniform and faced death in its service could not ultimately be anything less than a full-fledged citizen and it was going to be very hard to make citizens out of some Negroes without making citizens out of all.*[188]

Wherever they went, the Union soldiers were followed by swarms of ex-slaves, carrying their possessions on their backs, eager to sample their new freedom. The government tried to meet this influx by setting up refugee camps, forming labor battalions and, early in 1863, enlisting African Americans in the Union army. According to authors Simmons and Turner: "Black men were quickly put to work behind the lines, constructing fortifications, caring for livestock, and other manual labor required to maintain army life…It was obvious to some that these willing black men would make strong soldiers, soldiers with a burning commitment to establish their own freedom and the freedom of their brothers in bondage."[189]

The average Yankee soldier objected at first to any contact with African Americans. Yet by 1863, emancipation was a fact and the men soon adjusted to it. General Benjamin Butler, a staunch abolitionist, explained his extensive use of African American troops: "I knew that they would fight more desperately than any white troops in order to prevent capture, because they knew if captured they would be returned to slavery."[190]

While the two following accounts did not take place in Washington, D.C., they go to the issue of treatment of the soldiers and the threat they faced throughout the war in terms of their personal and medical safety.

Brigadier General A. Buford, besieging Columbus, Kentucky, sent the following note to his Federal opponent on April 13, 1864:

> *Fully capable of taking Columbus and its garrison by force, I desire to avoid the shedding of blood, and therefore demand the unconditional*

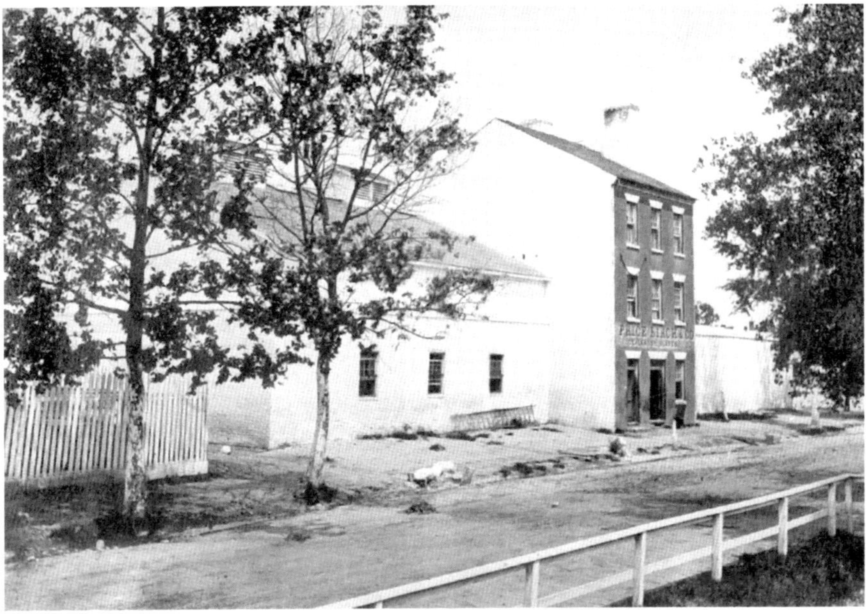

The Price, Birch and Company building, the slave trading firm, in 1862. *Courtesy of the Library of Congress, Washington, D.C.*

> *surrender of the forces under your command. Should you surrender, the Negroes now in arms will be returned to their masters. Should I however be compelled to take the place, no quarter will be shown to the Negro troops whatever; the white troops will be treated as prisoners of war.*[191]

A similar letter went from General J.B. Hood to the Union commander at Resaca, Georgia, on October 12, 1864.

> *I demand the immediate and unconditional surrender of the post and garrison under your command, and should this be acceded to all white officers and soldiers will be paroled in a few days. If the place is carried by assault, no prisoners will be taken...One not only may find instructions advising against the taking of Negro prisoners, and warnings that none would be taken, or, if taken that they would be killed; it is possible, also, to find clear evidence that these instructions and warnings were realized. Examples in addition to the Fort Pillow massacre exist. Before particularizing, however, attention is called to*

> *the fact that even the incomplete data of the adjutant general show twenty-one Negro soldiers as having been "killed after capture." That this is an underestimation will appear from the following material.*[192]

On September 2, 1863, the assistant adjutant general for Confederate general Johnston wrote to Colonel John Griffith that he had heard reports of the hanging or shooting by members of the latter's command of "certain federal prisoners and African Americans in arms at Jackson, Louisiana, on August 3 [1863]," and ordered him to investigate and give a report on the matter.

On September 2, 1863, Colonel Griffith answered:

> *In reply to your note just received I would say that a squad of African Americans was captured on or about the 3d of August, at Jackson, Louisiana. When the command started back, the Negroes, under guard, were ordered on in advance of the command, and learning that the guard had taken the wrong road, Colonel Powers and myself rode on in advance to put them in the proper route for camp. About the time we were reaching them, or shortly before, four of the Negroes attempted to escape. They were immediately fired into by the guard; this created some excitement, and a general stampede among them, whereupon the firing became general upon them from the guard, and few, I think, succeeded in making good their escape. There were no federal* [i.e. white] *prisoners among them, having been separated the night previous. No further particulars remembered. My own opinion is that the Negroes were summarily disposed of; by whom I cannot say…The whole transaction was contrary to my wishes, and against my own consent.*

This affair seems to have died with the endorsement, dated from Canton, Mississippi, on September 17, 1863, by Major General S.D. Lee, in forwarding the statements of the three colonels, that "I do not consider it to the interests of the service that this matter be further investigated at present. A Court of Inquiry or a Court-Martial will afford the only means of gaining correct information."[193]

According to several accounts from February 1864 of the First Mississippi during battle in Arkansas, the regiment was surrounded by enemy combatants. The story told was that the soldiers were captured and murdered, with fourteen being killed and six wounded. In March 1864, the Third United States Colored Cavalry reported that during a skirmish in Mississippi, sixteen of their soldiers were captured and put to death.[194] Other reports from regiments such as the Eighth United States Colored Heavy Artillery Regiment and the First Kansas confirmed such reports of violence and brutality against African American soldiers.[195]

The policy of the Confederate government of refusing to view captured African Americans as soldiers for prisoner of war purposes was extremely problematic for the Union army. Furthermore, as previously stated, it filled African American soldiers with a sense of the unknown that made engaging in battle that much more difficult.

Part of the issue for African American troops was proving their valor and themselves in battle. Fatigue duty was the harshest at the beginning of the war because of questions regarding whether the African American soldiers would fight and how valiantly they would fight. With this question summarily answered in the positive toward the end of the war, and with many African American troops proving themselves to be brave and courageous under fire, fatigue duties had lessened to certain extents.[196]

There were, though, certain African American regiments that were organized specifically for fatigue duty, and their sole purpose was to support the white troops with hard labor throughout the war effort.[197] There were seven "fatigue" African American regiments—the 42nd, 63rd, 64th, 69th, 101st, 123rd and 124th—but at least three of them ended up doing battle with Confederate troops.[198]

There were examples of such hard labor for African American troops that it seems to have had a direct bearing on fatalities in addition to being generally demoralizing, unpleasant and unhealthy.[199] Clear evidence exists demonstrating that African American troops were not equipped as well as others. Additionally, until the equalization of pay in June 1864, the clothing allowance for all African Americans came to thirty-six dollars per year while that for the lowest ranking whites equaled forty-two dollars. Moreover, frequent complaints arose from the African American troops that the hard labor and extraordinary hours of duty required of them prevented proper care of what clothing and equipment they did have, inadequate though it might have been.[200]

3

AFRICAN AMERICAN HEALTHCARE PROVIDERS IN D.C. DURING THE CIVIL WAR

During the war, there was a large demand for manual laborers in Washington, D.C. Contrabands could find work behind Union lines, doing everything from constructing fortifications around the city to seamstress work to nursing. According to author Robert Harrison:

> *In June 1862, the engineer in charge of the defense of Washington asked General James Wadsworth, the military governor in charge of the District, for a detail of "Contrabands to work...Wadsworth replied that there were only 100 contrabands under his direction and they were needed for hospital duties. By the middle of the war, over 300 contrabands were employed in military hospitals in Washington DC.*[201]

Through the exhaustive research of historian Lisa King, information regarding African American women who served in the navy as nurses is now available. King's research looks at the National Archives records, which, according to historian Mary Elizabeth Carnegie, shows that "these records kept on nurses at 11 hospitals in three states, 181 colored—men and women—served between July 16, 1863 and June 14, 1864; sixteen at the Convalescent Hospital, Baltimore Maryland; fourteen at the Contraband Hospital, Portsmouth, Virginia; three at the Flag of Truce Boat, from Fort Monroe, Virginia; forty-six at the Contraband Small Pox Hospital, New Bern, North Carolina; forty-six at Jarvis US G[eneral] Hospital, Baltimore, Maryland; twenty-one at Chesapeake

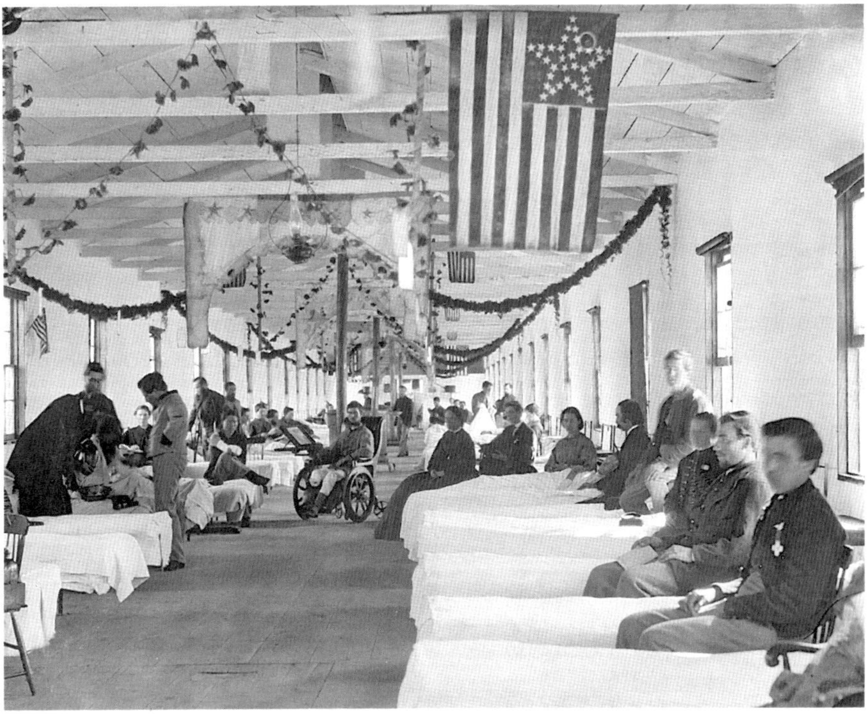

Carver Hospital, Washington, D.C. *Courtesy of the National Archives and Records Administration.*

Hospital, Virginia; one at Green Heights Hospital, Virginia; three at McKim's Mansion Hospital, near Alexandria, Virginia; and seven at Patterson Park, U.S. General Hospital Baltimore."[202]

On August 3, 1861, the War Department authorized each regiment to have one chaplain. There were no age limits or educational requirements for chaplains. They simply had to be ordained ministers of a Christian denomination. On July 17, 1862, in response to backlash from the Jewish community, the requirements of a chaplain were changed: "That no person shall be appointed a chaplain in the United States Army who is not a regularly ordained minister of some religious denomination and who does not present testimonials of his good standing…with a recommendation of his appointment as an army chaplain from some authorized ecclesiastical body, or not less than give accredited ministers belonging to said religious demonization." The role of chaplains was varied. While there were some fighting chaplains, the main scope of chaplain duties involved attending to the spiritual needs of soldiers, caring for the wounded, providing last rites, organizing funeral services, counseling soldiers, organizing temperance societies, teaching illiterate soldiers to reach and writing letters for wounded and dying soldiers.[203]

ALEXANDER AUGUSTA

In a letter to Secretary of War James J. Ferree, the commander of one of the D.C. contraband camps stated:

> *Knowing that Dr. Augusta ranked as major and that I ranked only as Captain, I felt at a loss as to assign to duty an officer who outranked me. I referred him to Dr. C.B. Webster, Surgeon in charge of the Contraband Camp Hospital, who being a contract surgeon was embarrassed by the same consideration.*[204]

The inherent difficulties that such a situation presented were not lost on Augusta.[205] His professionalism appears to have never been in question. In an order granting Augusta an eight-day leave on January 20, 1864, Brigadier General William Birney declared that "Surgeon Augusta has worked indefatigably" during his time at Camp Stanton.[206] Augusta met with President Lincoln in 1863. As recounted by his mentee Dr. Abbott:

> *The White House was ablaze of lights. Soldiers were guarding the entrance. Carriages containing handsomely dressed ladies, citizens and soldiers were continually depositing the elite of Washington at the entrance to the porch…Mr. Lincoln gave Augusta's hand a hearty shake and spoke to him. We then passed out into a room called…the East Room where we became the centre of attention…stares and fascinating* [sic] *eyes leveled at us for half an hour or so.*[207]

Augusta's performance, on the other hand, was not enough to overcome some of the innate prejudice that he faced. For example, he was assigned to the Seventh United States Colored Infantry and went with it into garrison at Camp Stanton, near Bryantown, Maryland. He was the senior surgeon when in February 1864, the two white assistant surgeons, as well as the surgeons and assistant surgeons of the Ninth and Nineteenth Regiments, addressed a letter to Abraham Lincoln:

> *When we made application for position on the Colored Service, the understanding was universal that all commissioned officers were to be white men. Judge of our surprise when, upon joining our respective regiments, we found that the Senior Surgeon of the Command was an African American. We claim to be behind no one, in a desire for the elevation and improvement of the colored race in this Country, and we are willing to sacrifice much in so grand a cause, as our present positions may testify. But we cannot in any cause, willingly compromise what we consider a proper self-respect; nor do we deem that the interests of either the country or of the colored race, can demand this of us. Such degradation, we believed to be involved in our voluntarily continuing in the service, as subordinate to a colored officer. We therefore most respectfully, yet earnestly, request that this unexpected, unusual, and most unpleasant relationship in which we have been placed, may in some way be terminated.*[208]

Augusta would also be subject to several instances of overt racism. Augusta would continue to suffer such indignities at the hands of fellow officers for his entire career. With respect to his pay, the year after being commissioned, Augusta informed Senator Henry Wilson that the army paymaster was paying him only seven dollars per month.[209] This was significantly less than white officers of his rank. Because of the times in which Augusta lived, he tried to obliterate discrimination when he found himself confronted with such blatant intolerance and bigotry as described above.[210]

A prime example is this: Traveling to testify in a court-martial on February 1, 1864, Augusta was delayed due to a trolley car incident. Documenting the reason for his lateness in a letter to the judge advocate, Augusta wrote: "I have been obstructed in getting to the court this morning by the conductor of Car No. 32 of the 14th Street line of the city railway." He hailed a car on Fourteenth Street, and when he tried to enter the car, the conductor stopped him and informed him that he had to ride in the front of the car. When Augusta refused to ride at all, the conductor rejected him from the car platform, thus, forcing Augusta to travel to court on foot in the mud and rain.

Augusta wrote a letter to the assistant secretary of war about the incident, stating that he was detained in the court case because of the "outrage" committed by the conductor of Car Number Thirty-two of the D.C. City Railway. Dr. Anderson Abbott wrote about the incident, portraying Augusta as something of a civil rights hero.

On reaching the court on foot, Augusta gave a statement to the judge advocate as to why he was late and the incident that had occurred on the railway. He also wrote to Senator Sumner of Massachusetts.[211]

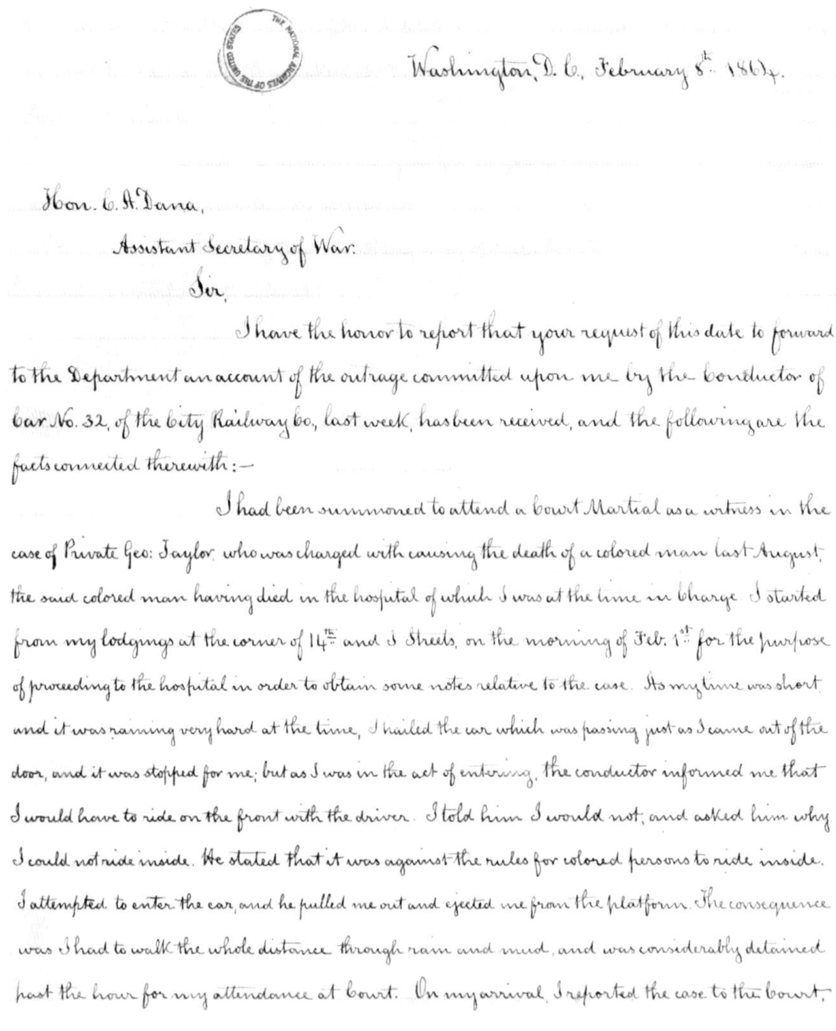

Washington, D.C., February 8th 1864.

Hon. C. A. Dana,
Assistant Secretary of War.
Sir,

I have the honor to report that your request of this date to forward to the Department an account of the outrage committed upon me by the Conductor of Car No. 32, of the City Railway Co., last week, has been received, and the following are the facts connected therewith:—

I had been summoned to attend a Court Martial as a witness in the case of Private Geo: Taylor, who was charged with causing the death of a colored man last August, the said colored man having died in the hospital of which I was at the time in Charge. I started from my lodgings at the corner of 14th and I Streets, on the morning of Feb. 1st for the purpose of proceeding to the hospital in order to obtain some notes relative to the case. As my time was short, and it was raining very hard at the time, I hailed the car which was passing just as I came out of the door, and it was stopped for me; but as I was in the act of entering, the conductor informed me that I would have to ride on the front with the driver. I told him I would not, and asked him why I could not ride inside. He stated that it was against the rules for colored persons to ride inside. I attempted to enter the car, and he pulled me out and ejected me from the platform. The consequence was I had to walk the whole distance through rain and mud, and was considerably detained past the hour for my attendance at Court. On my arrival, I reported the case to the Court,

A letter written by Dr. Alexander Augusta to Assistant Secretary of War Charles A. Dana regarding the street car incident. *Courtesy of the National Archives and Records Administration.*

In his book *The African American's Civil War*, historian James McPherson summed up the positive results of this negative experience, saying: "Augusta's letter added a strong impetus to Sumner's antisegregation drive. Sumner read it into the *Congressional Globe* and introduced a resolution instructing the Senate District of Columbia Committee to frame a law barring street car discrimination in the district."[212]

The bigotry that Augusta and other African Americans serving during the Civil War shared was not an experience encountered by their white counterparts and therefore was not something that these individuals could completely understand. Many white soldiers were dealing with overcoming their own prejudices regarding African Americans. And in the middle of a traumatic war, it was often a difficult hurdle to climb.

Finally, as with many African American volunteers in the Union army, Augusta had great difficulty collecting the salary commensurate with his rank. The paymaster in Baltimore, Maryland, insisted that Augusta should be paid seven dollars per month. This was vastly under what someone of Augusta's rank should have been paid. As he had done all of his life, Augusta stood up for his rights and fought for the pay due to him, rejecting the injustice of a lower salary.[213] Following a letter from Senator Henry Wilson to Secretary of War Edwin M. Stanton and an order from Stanton to the paymaster general, after fifty-three weeks Major Augusta was compensated according to his rank.[214]

Friends and foes alike saw Augusta as a fighter and champion for the rights of African Americans. As Newby puts it: "In his admiration of his mentor and colleague, Dr. Alexander T. Augusta, Abbott at the same time questioned the actions of Augusta when Augusta openly challenged a system which suppressed the advancement of his race." Augusta had worked hard for his position in society and insisted that his freedom, not condescension or favor, should give him the rights accorded to any other free citizen in the United States. He did not hesitate to challenge those who stood in his way.[215]

According to Augusta, while traveling from the Baltimore/D.C. area to Philadelphia during the war, he was attacked by two men who tore off his officer's insignia. An angry mob then gathered and threatened his life. Augusta was saved by a couple of provost guards; however, soon after this, Augusta was accosted by another man who stepped in front of him and punched him in the face. This man was arrested, and Augusta finally made his way to his train, meeting up with Major General Joseph Hooker's staff, who agreed to accompany Augusta to Philadelphia to protect him from more harm. While Augusta "had always known Baltimore as a place where it is considered a virtue to mob colored people," the entire incident was terribly demoralizing for Augusta. According to Augusta, "I had only volunteered to bind up the wounds of those colored men who should volunteer, as well as those rebels and copperheads that the fortune of war might throw into my hands."[216]

Anderson Abbott

Anderson Abbott's first letter of application to serve in the Civil War was dated February 4, 1863, and was addressed to Edwin M. Stanton:

> *Dear Sir. I learn by our city papers that it is the intention of the United States government to raise 150,000 colored troops. Being one of the class of persons, I beg to apply for a commission as Assistant Surgeon. My qualifications are: that I am twenty-five years of age, I have been engaged in the study of practice of medicine five years; I am a licentiate of the College of Physicians and Surgeons Upper Canada—a board of examiners appointed by the Governor General to examine candidates for license to practice. I am also a matriculant of the Toronto University. It is my intention to go up for my degree of "Bachelor of Medicine" in the spring.*[217]

After writing this letter to Stanton in February 1863 and receiving no response, Abbott again wrote to Stanton after his mentor, Alexander Augusta, received his commission:

> *Sir: I beg most respectfully to apply for a situation as Medical Cadet in the army. I am a coloured man, and would desire to be appointed in one of the coloured regiments, if you think favorably on my application. It may be some recommendation to add that I have been a pupil of Dr. A.T. Augusta for several years. He received a commission from you, as surgeon, recently. He will give you all the information you may require concerning my character and attainments.*[218]

It would be several more months before Abbott would get his appointment, but eventually he was stationed at Freedmen's Hospital in Washington, D.C., the former Contraband Hospital, with his mentor Augusta. Historians also point to Jerome R. Riley, author of *The Philosophy of Negro Suffrage* and an African Canadian like Abbott, as joining Abbott and Augusta at the hospital and working in Washington, D.C., at the hospital after the war.[219] Riley would later go on to graduate from Howard University's Medical School in 1873. Freedmen's Hospital was established in 1863 in order to provide care and training to African Americans. Alexander Augusta served as head of the hospital from 1863 to 1864, followed by William Powell and Anderson Abbott. According to Dr. Robert Reyburn, surgeon in chief of Freedmen's Hospital from 1868 to 1875: "Washington during the war was the haven of refuse for [African Americans]; the sick, the infirm and destitute among them felt that if they could but reach Washington, they would be cared for and all their wants would be supplied."[220]

Dr. Abbott eventually became an acting assistant surgeon to the United States.[221] He worked at the Contraband Hospital in Washington, D.C. Abbott was contracted to receive $80 per month on June 26, 1863, and by February 26, 1864, he was receiving $100 per month. Dr. Abbott was on duty in Washington, D.C., from June 26, 1863, to June 25, 1864.

The road that African Americans traveled in order to participate in the Civil War was difficult. Prior to May 1861, slaves who escaped from their masters would be returned if caught. This practice changed with General Benjamin F. Butler who, rather than returning three slaves to their owners, labeled the slaves "contrabands"—possessions confiscated as the result of a war with a foreign government. This led to a flood of slaves escaping to northern camps in hope of making a better life for themselves. Anderson Abbott was a medical officer in charge of such a camp, which unfortunately had inadequate supplies, deteriorating conditions and more people than the camp had the capacity to handle.[222]

Historian Newby tells the story of a riot that erupted—in part because of the Draft Law, which allowed a draftee up to $300 toward a substitute draftee—additionally, because African Americans were exempt from the draft, poor whites began to riot in New York and Boston. According to Abbott, who was in New York with Augusta's wife while traveling to Washington, D.C., to meet up with Augusta:

> *I followed Dr. Augusta on the 10th of July, 1863. Mrs. Augusta and myself started on that day for Washington and here I must mention an incident which occurred at the Depot in NY while we were waiting for a train. We arrived in NY about dusk and found that our train would not start until 10 o'clock that night. While Mrs. Augusta and I were standing in the depot a man came pretending to be drunk, fell up against Mrs. Augusta. I pushed him off. He then approached me with a threatening attitude but did not dare to strike me. After indulging in considerable violent language and profanity he went out and brought in a big Irish man who began to abuse us in the coarsest language threatening to stamp our lives out and do many other dreadful things. We looked around for a policeman to protect us. There was not a soul to be seen about the place but these two drunken thugs and a man who appeared to be a watchman employed by the ferry company. We asked him if there were no*

> *means by which we could receive protection. He did not deign to answer us or notice us in any way. At this juncture several soldiers came in the room. They seemed to have consorted with these two men because they addressed them by name and seemed to be endeavoring to coax these partners to go out with them. Mrs. Augusta and myself thought it a good opportunity escape.*[223]

Abbott tells a fascinating story in an article entitled "Colored Female Corporal" about Corporal Rogers, a former slave who, when the Civil War commenced, was coached by a Union spy detained on the property of her master to head for the Union lines. She took the advice, using a Federal soldier's uniform given to her by the spy as her means of camouflage. She was a member of the USCT when Abbott met her. Abbott described her and the meeting as follows:

> *Your correspondent first met Corporal Rogers in the hospital at Washington, DC where she had been admitted and was suffering from epileptic fits. She appeared to be a woman of about thirty years of age, 5 feet 7 inches in height, light grey eyes, light complexion, a masculine cast of countenance, and with her hair parted on the side. She convinced the writer that she could carry out the deception very successfully, she could also shoulder a musket and go through the "manual" with the precision and dexterity of a veteran.*[224]

WILLIS REVELS

Willis Revels was a member of the Twenty-eighth USCT and a reverend as well as a physician. He was also the chief recruiting officer for the regiment. The regiment was one of the units responsible for defending Washington, D.C. Recruits of the regiment trained for three months in Indianapolis and then, on April 25, 1863, traveled to Washington, D.C.[225]

WILLIAM POWELL

Dr. William R. Powell was the son of an African American physician from New York. Although there is not a great deal of evidence regarding his education, it appears that he was in England before the war and received his medical degree from the College of Physicians and Surgeons in London.

He began serving in the war on September 1, 1864, as chief surgeon, being mustered out of battalion on October 20, 1865, and serving at the Contraband Hospital in Washington, D.C. Powell appears to have had some difficulties while serving during the war. As described by Anderson Abbott:

> *On June 26th I* [Abbott] *was commissioned and placed on duty in the same hospital under Dr. Augusta who was surgeon in charge. He had one assistant a Dr. Wm. Powell, a graduate of College Phy. Surgeon, England. The hospital contained a capacity of 300 beds. It was used for the treatment of Freedmen and Colored soldiers. It was fully equipped with a competent staff of nurses, laundry women, cooks, stewards and clerks, etc. and was situated about 3 miles from Washington. Hospitals were established for colored troops and Indians in every military district but towards the close of the war colored troops were sent to the hospital that was most convenient. A few months after Dr. Augusta was sent to Camp Birney, as before intimated, Dr. Powell was suspended and cashiered. And the following November I was placed in charge and continued in charge of Hospital until I resigned and returned home in 1866 after the close of the war.*[226]

Martin Delany

A physician who occupies a unique space in the lexicon of African American physicians during the Civil War is Dr. Martin Robison Delany. Delany was an abolitionist, physician, colleague and friend to Frederick Douglass. He spent a great deal of time abroad championing the Black Nationalism movement. He was abroad when the Civil War broke out and came back to the United States in 1861 to champion the cause of African American soldiers fighting in the Civil War.[227] When the Fifty-fourth Massachusetts Volunteer Infantry was mustered in 1863, commanded by Robert Gould Shaw, Delany was ready to serve.

Delany did not serve as a physician during the war, but he was a doctor nonetheless and had a fascinating path to serving in the Civil War. In 1861, he returned to the United States, after traveling to Liberia and England, to champion the cause of African American soldiers fighting in the Civil War. Delany was something of a renaissance man during the war, acting as a recruiter (in D.C.) and in 1865 being commissioned a major of infantry as well as being a physician.[228]

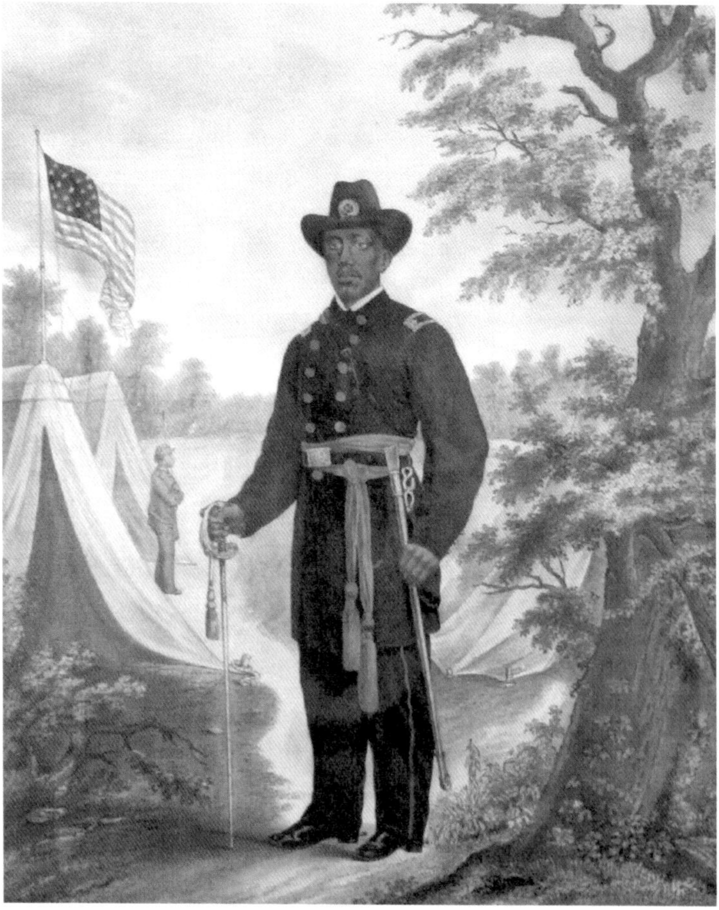

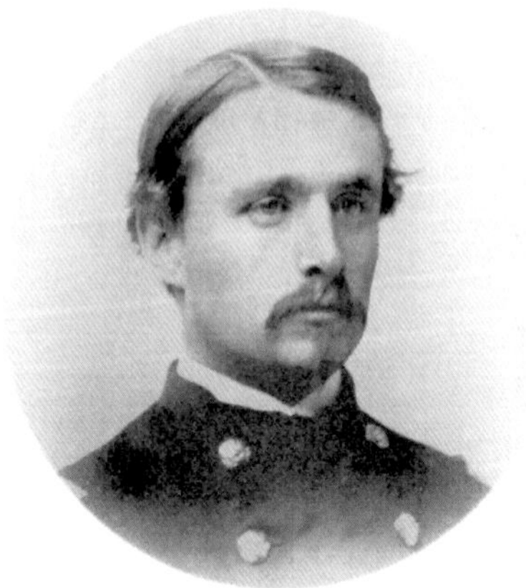

Above: Major Martin Delany. *Courtesy of the National Portrait Gallery, Smithsonian Institution.*

Right: Robert Gould Shaw. *Courtesy of the Houghton Library Collections, Harvard College Library.*

HENRY TURNER

Fourteen African American chaplains served as commissioned officers during the Civil War. There was a great push on the part of both African Americans and abolitionists to have commissioned officers serve in the war effort.[229] Secretary of War Stanton had decreed that only white officers would be commissioned officers in USCT and other African American regiments. Governor Andrew of Massachusetts worked with the War Department to identify a group of African Americans who could be commissioned.

The duties of a wartime chaplain were far reaching and varied and included healthcare and medical duties. Chaplains were often called on to visit the wounded and ill in camp hospitals, take on other healthcare roles and aid in burying those who died. There were fourteen African American clergymen who served as Union army chaplains who should be noted for their care of African Americans during the war. Henry McNeal Turner—who also served as a journalist and writer—was one of the fourteen.[230] He served as a chaplain for the First USCT based out of D.C.

HARRIET TUBMAN

Harriet Tubman was a nurse in Port Royal and aided the majority of soldiers, who had dysentery and smallpox. While she was receiving government remuneration, she eventually agreed to replace the money she received from the government in place of money she made selling pies and root beer. After the Emancipation Proclamation passed in January 1863, Tubman was dedicated to the war. She led a band of scouts through the land around Port Royal. Tubman also worked with Secretary of War Edwin Stanton in Washington, D.C., as well as Colonel James Montgomery, to put her knowledge of the terrain to positive use for the war effort.

SOJOURNER TRUTH

Sojourner Truth was known as a champion for the rights of women and African Americans and worked in the Freedmen's Hospital and Freedmen's Village to bring comfort to the soldiers during the war.[231]

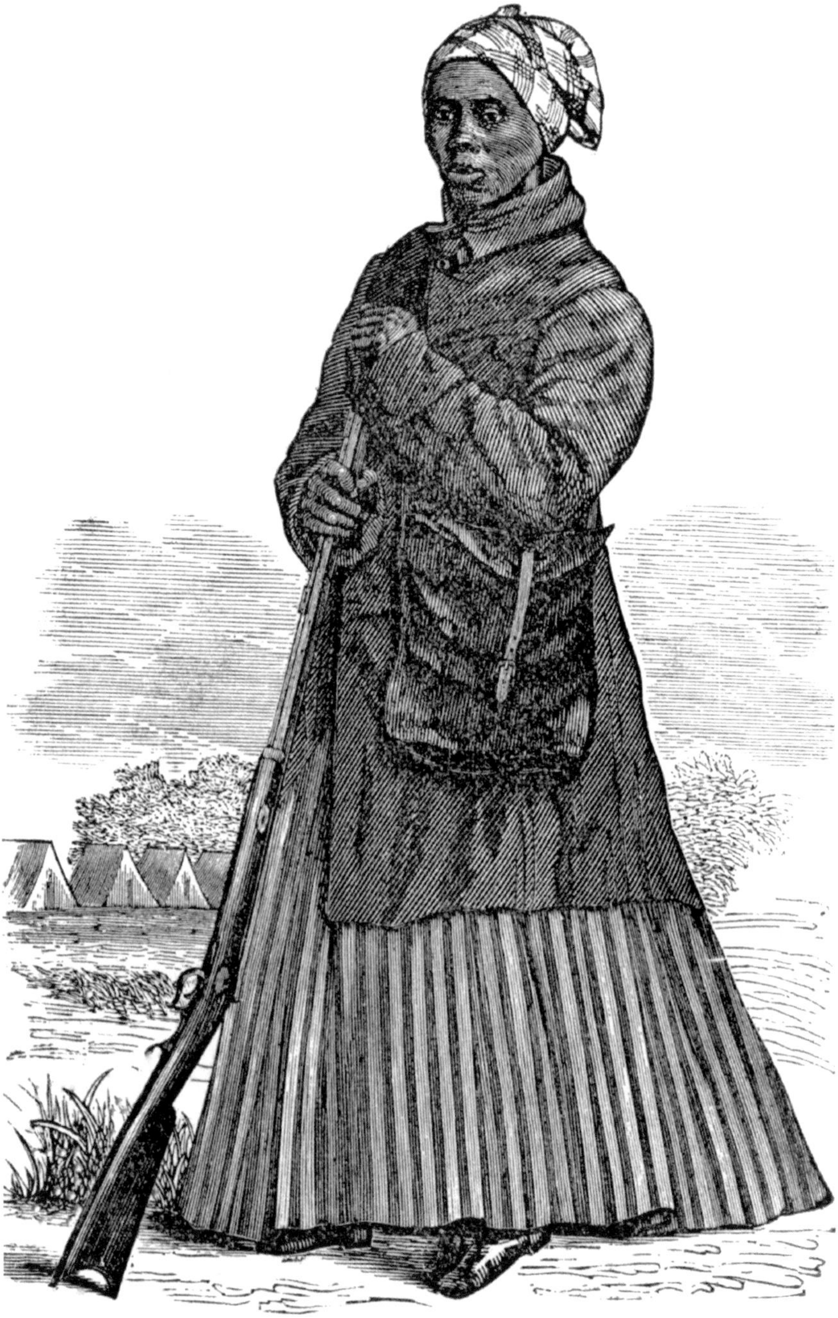

Harriet Tubman. *Courtesy of the National Portrait Gallery, Smithsonian Institution.*

Sojourner Truth followed the Civil War closely at the point when thousands of enslaved African Americans began making their way to Washington, D.C. In June 1864, Truth started a book tour that took her to Detroit, Boston and ultimately, Washington, D.C. Truth was also interested in meeting with President Lincoln. With the help of Mary Todd's confidante Elizabeth Keckley, the meeting was set up. Truth wanted to speak with Lincoln about the treatment of African Americans in the contraband camps.[232] In a letter written to friend Rowland Johnson, Truth speaks about the meeting:

> *It was about 8 o'clock a.m., when I called on the President. Upon entering his reception room we found about a dozen persons in waiting, among them two colored women. I had quite a pleasant time waiting until he was disengaged, and enjoyed his conversation with others. He showed as much kindness and consideration to the colored persons as to the whites…The President was seated at his desk. Mrs. C*[olman] *said to him, "This is Sojourner Truth, who has come all the way from Michigan to see you." He then rose, gave me his hand, made a bow, and said, "I am pleased to see you."…As I was taking my leave, he arose and took my hand, and said he would be pleased to have me call again. I felt that I was in the presence of a friend, and I now thank God from the bottom of my heart that I always have advocated his causes, and have done it openly and boldly. I shall feel still more in duty bound to do so in time to come. May God assist me.*[233]

Like Alexander Augusta, Sojourner Truth also fought for equality on street cars. Even through Truth advocated to President Lincoln, who signed the law banning street car segregation on March 3, 1865, Truth still faced difficulties traveling in and around D.C. On one particular occasion, Truth boarded a streetcar with a nurse heading to Freedmen's Hospital when fellow white passengers complained about having to share the care with Truth and her companion. On another occasion, traveling to Freedmen's Hospital with abolitionist and inspector of hospitals Laura Haviland with supplies for patients, Truth described the following when she and Haviland attempted to board a streetcar:

> *The conductor pushed me back, saying "Get out of the way and let this lady (Haviland) come in." "Whoop" said I, "I am a lady too."…A lady saw some colored women looking wistfully toward a car, when the conductor, halting, said, "Walk in ladies," Now they who had so lately cursed me for wanting to ride, could stop for black as well as white, and could even condescend to say, "Walk in, ladies."*

Jane Isabella Saunders

Jane Isabella Saunders, also known as "Aunt Jane," was hired by Alexander T. Augusta at the Contraband Hospital in D.C. to tend to the sick and injured. She worked at the hospital through 1865 and stated, "There were always two of us in each ward, and we had to make the beds, and keep the ward clean, besides wait on the sick...Many a night I had to sit up all night to wait on the sick, give them medicine or food, and to help take care of them in every way that was needed."[234]

Maria Toliver

Maria Toliver was born in 1839 on a plantation in Williamsburg. She fled to Washington in 1862 According to Toliver, in her pension application, "I was born in Williamsburg, Virginia and was sold into King William Col., VA and ran off from my master about 1862…about 3 months after I came here to Washington, I [was] hired to a Dr. James Pettijohn to nurse in the Hospital at Camp Barker."[235] She would later meet and marry her husband at the hospital, and they would go on to work together after the war at Freedmen's Hospital.[236]

Maria Mitchell

Maria Mitchell was an ex-slave who served in several hospitals in and around Washington and Alexandra Virginia, including L'Ouverture Hospital and the Contraband Hospital. She contracted with the army on May 16, 1864, to serve as a nurse.[237]

There are some accounts of these hospitals. The National Archives lists the employees of "the hospital at the corner of Washington and Wolfe streets as: Harriet Graves, McAllister and Matilda Craig, William Lowe, Peter Willis, Ann Jones, Maria Mitchell, Phoebe Ann Turner, and possibly John Naylor."[238] Mitchell did a great deal of the cooking duties. Matilda Yates Craig married McAllister Craig who would go on to enlist in the Thirty-first USCI.[239]

ALPHEUS TUCKER

Alpheus Tucker was a Michigan native. He was born in Detroit in the mid-1840s and grew up in Toledo, Ohio, before attending Oberlin College. He graduated from the Iowa College of Physicians and Surgeons in 1865. Like several of his counterparts, he also served in the Contraband Hospital in Washington, D.C., and remained in D.C. after the war.

CORTLANDT VAN RENSSELAER CREED

Dr. Cortlandt Van Rensselaer Creed entered Yale University School of Medicine in 1854. Finishing his studies in 1857, he was the first African American to graduate from Yale's Medical School. When the Civil War commenced, Dr. Creed repeatedly contacted the Connecticut governor requesting a commission in the army. Once the army began actively recruiting African American soldiers in 1863, Creed was given a commission in the service, appointed in 1864 as acting surgeon of the Thirtieth Connecticut Colored Volunteer Infantry. [240] This was eight years after the Connecticut Assembly removed all references to race from the state constitution. Dr. Creed's thesis was entitled "On the Blood." The Thirtieth Regiment would eventually merge with the Thirty-First Connecticut in June 1864. Creed's regiment stayed around D.C., in Annapolis and Viriginia. The regiments collectively totaled 1,700 men and suffered 600 casualties.[241]

JOHN RAPIER

Dr. John Rapier Jr. was an acting assistant surgeon in Freedmen's Hospital in D.C. toward the end of the war. He was born in Alabama and received his medical degree in Iowa from Keokuk Medical College in 1864.[242] In a letter dated August 19, 1864, from Rapier, who was stationed at Freedmen's Hospital, to his uncle James P. Thomas, Rapier speaks about his time in the war:

> *I am always glad to hear from you and our St. Louis friends, but I am a little afraid I will be considered as a very poor correspondent after a*

while, on account of the few letters I write. Indeed Uncle James I never worked so hard, and had so little rest, and felt so tired at night as I do now. Of my success and failures, for I have both, it does not become me to speak, for your satisfaction and of those others who kindly feel an interest in me and my welfare I may venture to say that my mentality… so far stands approved by the Med. Director of the Department to whom I make daily, weekly, monthly and quarterly reports. There are many ladies here from the East, blessed old Massachusetts always in the lead of good works engaged in teaching and general supervision of the interest of the Freedmen in this City. They are a class the most indefatigable and earnest laborers I have ever seen engaged in any cause—wind, rain and storm never stop them—night and day these Angels of Mercy may be found engaged in the miserable filthy hovels of these poor people doing the most servile and menial duties. Foremost and bravest of these is a Miss Harriette Carter of Mass. Do not imagine Miss Carter to be an old and homely "one" who has…for someone to love for many years in vain, and has when up this occupation, perhaps as a penance for youthful indiscretion is saying "no" when somebody thought she ought to have said "yes." By no means—Miss Carter is 24 with rosy cheeks, pretty eyes and…the softest brown hair you ever felt, and as fully of learning as an Episcopal Minister or a Catholic Priest and would make even Henry Green laugh at her humor and wit. She is never seen with a sober face. And in making my daily rounds, I always encounter her, and have a half…pleasant chat before I assume the duties of the day. I have but little time to visit and therefore have but few acquaintances, and these poorly cultivated. I am socially speaking a "stick" and have but little pleasure as you know in making new friends. I much rather presume upon those I know. In our Hospital some changes have taken place. Surg. Horner (white) supersedes Surg. Powell (colo). The change was for the…services and I believe complexion had nothing to do with it. Surg. Horner is a skillful and well educated surg, and polite agreeable gentleman. Dr. Powell is retained as Asst. I have thought of resigning in Oct. for the purpose of attending lectures in the University of Harvard in Boston and trying for a Surgeon's Post in the spring. Perhaps I may, perhaps I may not give up this idea—I am undecided. On the 14th the most eventful event of my life occurred—I drew $100 less war tax $2.50 for Medical Services rendered the U.S. government. My draft was in favour of "Acting Asst. Surgeon Rank 1st Lieut. U.S.A." I read the *address several times—I liked it tho' I confess it read strange to me. In the spring I want my drafts payable to Maj. John H. Rapier Surg. U.S.A. I do not like the U.S. Service. However half loaf is better than no loaf. It is better to have a blue coat than no military coat. I would rather have the Mexican Green or English Purple. But I must tell you coloured men in the U.S. Uniform are much respect here, and in visiting the various Departments if the dress is that of an Officer, you receive the military salute from the ground as promptly as if your blood was Howard or Plantagenet instead of a Pompey or Cuffee's. I had decided not to wear the uniform but I have altered my mind—I shall appear hereafter in full dress gold lace, pointed hat, straps and all. Mr. Fred Douglass spoke here last night to an immense audience and today the President sent for him to visit him in the Capitol. Did you ever hear such nonsense?...I have been invited to take supper with Mr. Douglass tonight. I am proud of it. He visited the Hospital today. He is a fine looking gentleman. He made a fine impression on the public. I exceedingly regret to hear of Miss Virginia's ill health and hope she may be well soon. I shall write to Miss Pauline in a few days to whom make my apologies for not writing earlier. I have an opening here for Lady teacher. Pay depends on her qualifications. It may be $50 or $30 per month. If I had the money I would send for Sarah—I believe she could get $50. If you go to New York come by Washington if you can. I am sorry I have not money in my pocket to offer you a big time. But wait until September 30th and I will do the "clean thing" by you. In all Washington there is not a number one place for a Col. Gentleman to stop. But I will "fix" you up—if you give me "due and timely" notice. Write to me. Direct my letters John H. Rapier, M.D. Actg. Asst. Surg. U.S.A. Tell Mrs. Bailey I have written to her. Remember me to Mr. Clamorgan and the Johnsons, Mrs. Pritchard and Mr. Pritchard. Write soon. I am as usual yours, John Jr.*[243]

CHARLES PURVIS

Dr. Charles Purvis was the grandson of James Forten Sr., the civil rights leader. Purvis went to Oberlin College and attended Wooster Medical College. In 1864, Purvis began working as a military nurse at Camp Barker with ex-slaves. He graduated from medical school in 1865 and enlisted in

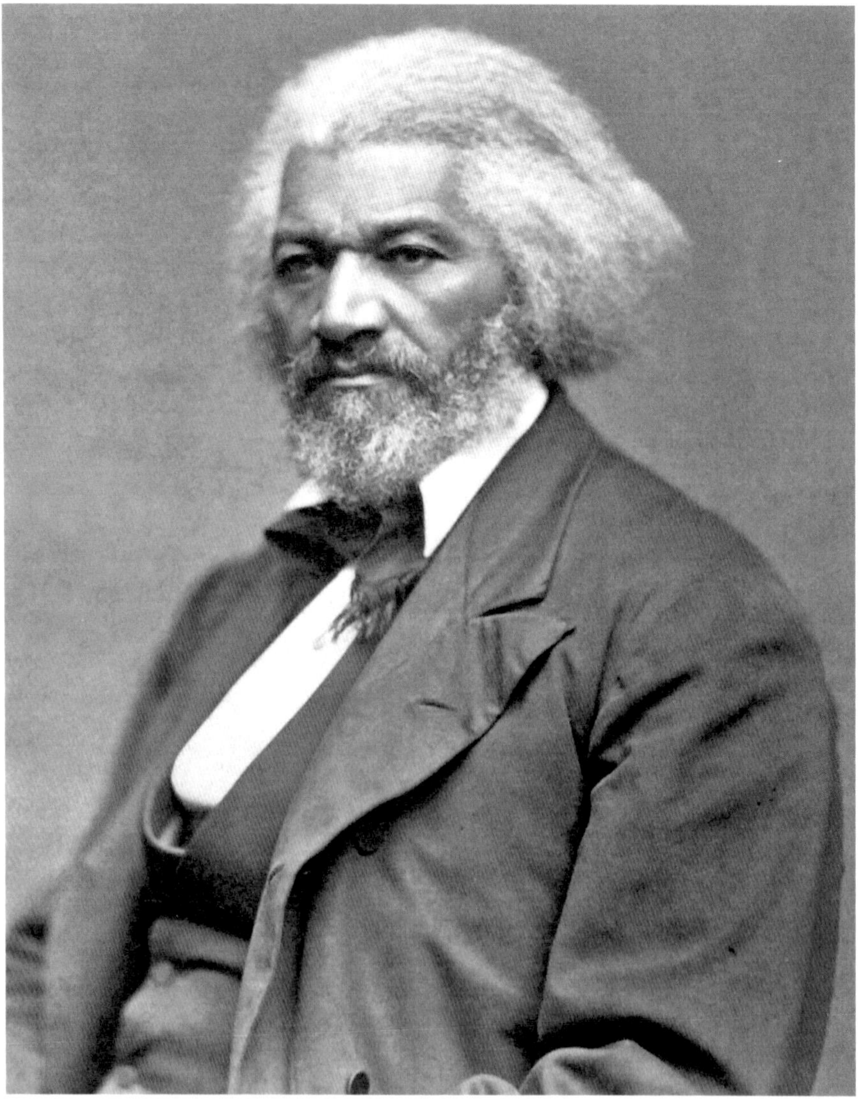

Frederick Douglass. *Courtesy of the National Archives and Records Administration.*

Opposite: Dr. Charles Burleigh Purvis. *Courtesy of the National Library of Medicine.*

the Union army as an acting assistant surgeon. He would serve from 1865 to 1869, treating mostly freedmen. While at the Freedmen's Hospital, Purvis saw a succession of leaders including Alexander Augusta, William Powell, Caleb Horn and Anderson Abbott.[244]

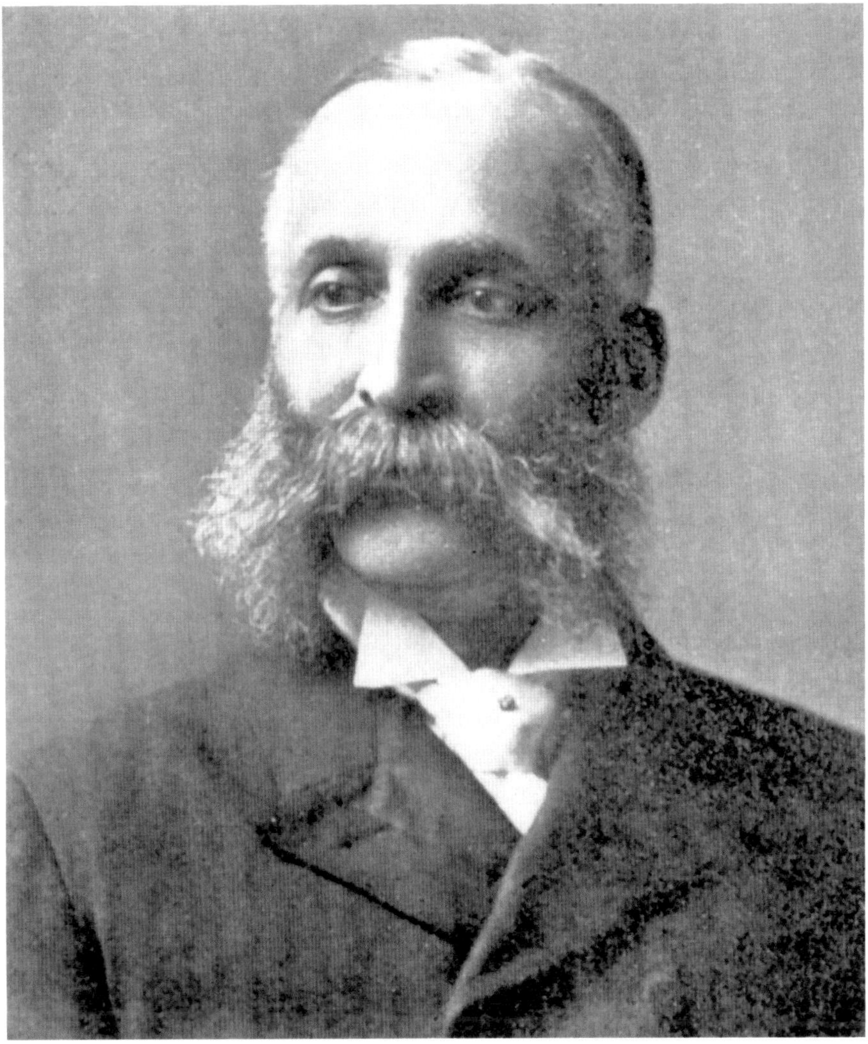

Purvis's thoughts on African Americans and their role in the Civil War were clear: "The Negro slave, guided by some altruistic power, embraced every opportunity to escape his bondage to the seat of government. He was not encouraged in his endeavor, really not desired, still in numbers he came."[245]

4

African American Healthcare in D.C. after the Civil War

Much of the behavioral issues that superior officers saw in soldiers may also be attributable to what we currently think of as post-traumatic stress disorder. According to Sara A.M. Ford of Kutztown University of Pennsylvania, "Data compiled from diaries and letters will affirm the presence of psychological disorders in soldiers who fought in the war. From this body of evidence, it is clear that soldiers of the American Civil War did indeed suffer from post-traumatic stress disorder and other psychological disorders."[246]

Saint Elizabeth's Hospital in southeast Washington, D.C., authorized in 1855, was originally called the Government Hospital for the Insane and was actively used during the Civil War. Union and Confederate soldiers, sailors and marines—including African-American troops—were treated at the hospital. President Abraham Lincoln, a frequent visitor to the hospital, noted that the many casualties created by the war often resulted in overcrowding at the hospital. Tents were erected behind the hospital to handle the overflow of combat casualties.

In 1865, with so many veterans needing long-term care, Lincoln appealed to Congress and the nation in his second inaugural address "to care for him who shall have borne the battle, and for his widow and his orphan." Those words later became the motto of the Veterans Administration, which became the Department of Veterans Affairs in 1989. Lincoln's efforts resulted in creation of the National Asylum for Disabled Volunteer Soldiers (NHDVS) in March 1865, which established a national government home for veterans of the Union's volunteer forces. A

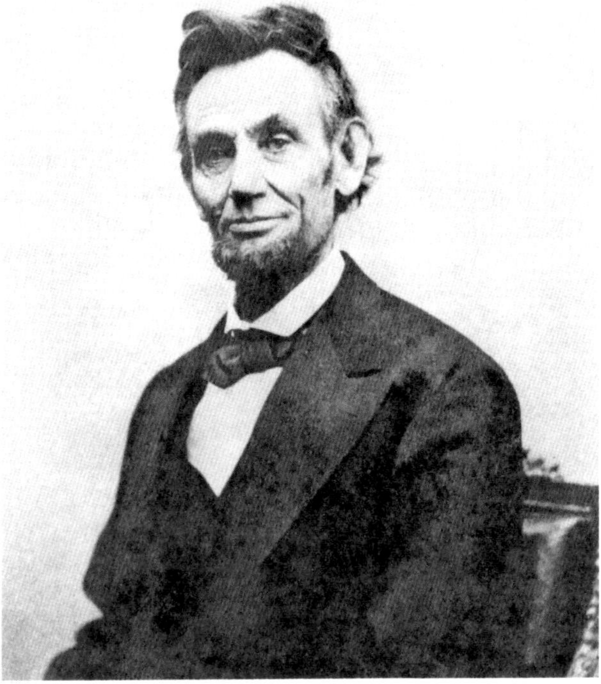

Left: President Abraham Lincoln. *Courtesy of the Library of Congress, Washington, D.C.*

Below: Ex-slaves attend a reunion in Washington, D.C. *Courtesy of the Library of Congress, Washington, D.C.*

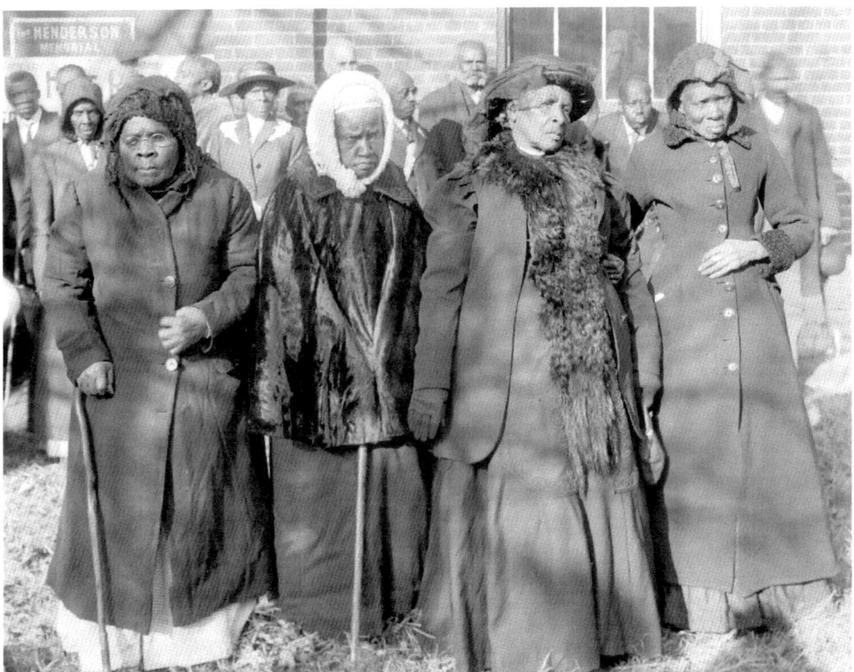

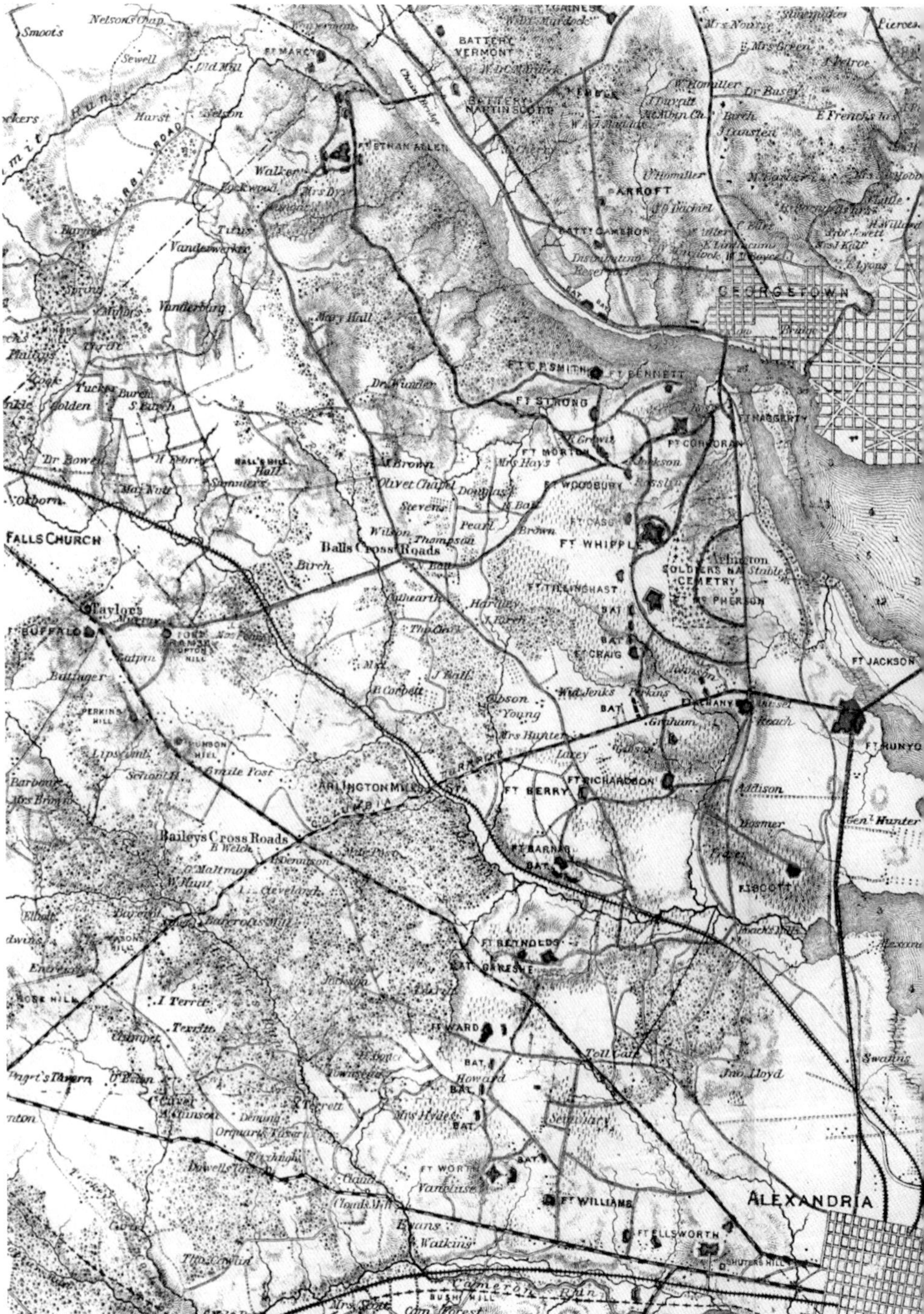
BATTERY VERMONT
BATTERY MARTIN SCOTT
FT MARCY
FT ETHAN ALLEN
Smoots
Sewell
Old Mill
KIRBY ROAD
Walker
Vanderwerker
Vanderburg
Mary Hall
Dr Wunder
GEORGETOWN
FT C.F. SMITH
FT BENNETT
FT STRONG
FT HAGGERTY
FT CORCORAN
FT MORTON
FT WOODBURY
FT CASS
FT WHIPPLE
FT TILLINGHAST
FT CRAIG
SOLDIERS NA CEMETERY
Olivet Chapel
Stevens
Thompson
Balls Cross Roads
FALLS CHURCH
Taylors
FT BUFFALO
FT JACKSON
FT RUNYON
Mrs Hunter
FT BERRY
FT RICHARDSON
ARLINGTON MILLS
Baileys Cross Roads
Addison
Gen.l Hunter
FT BARNARD
FT SCOTT
FT REYNOLDS
FT WARD
Toll Gate
Jno. Lloyd
Seminary
FT WORTH
FT WILLIAMS
FT ELLSWORTH
ALEXANDRIA
Clouds Mill
Evans
Watkins
BUSH HILL
Cameron Run

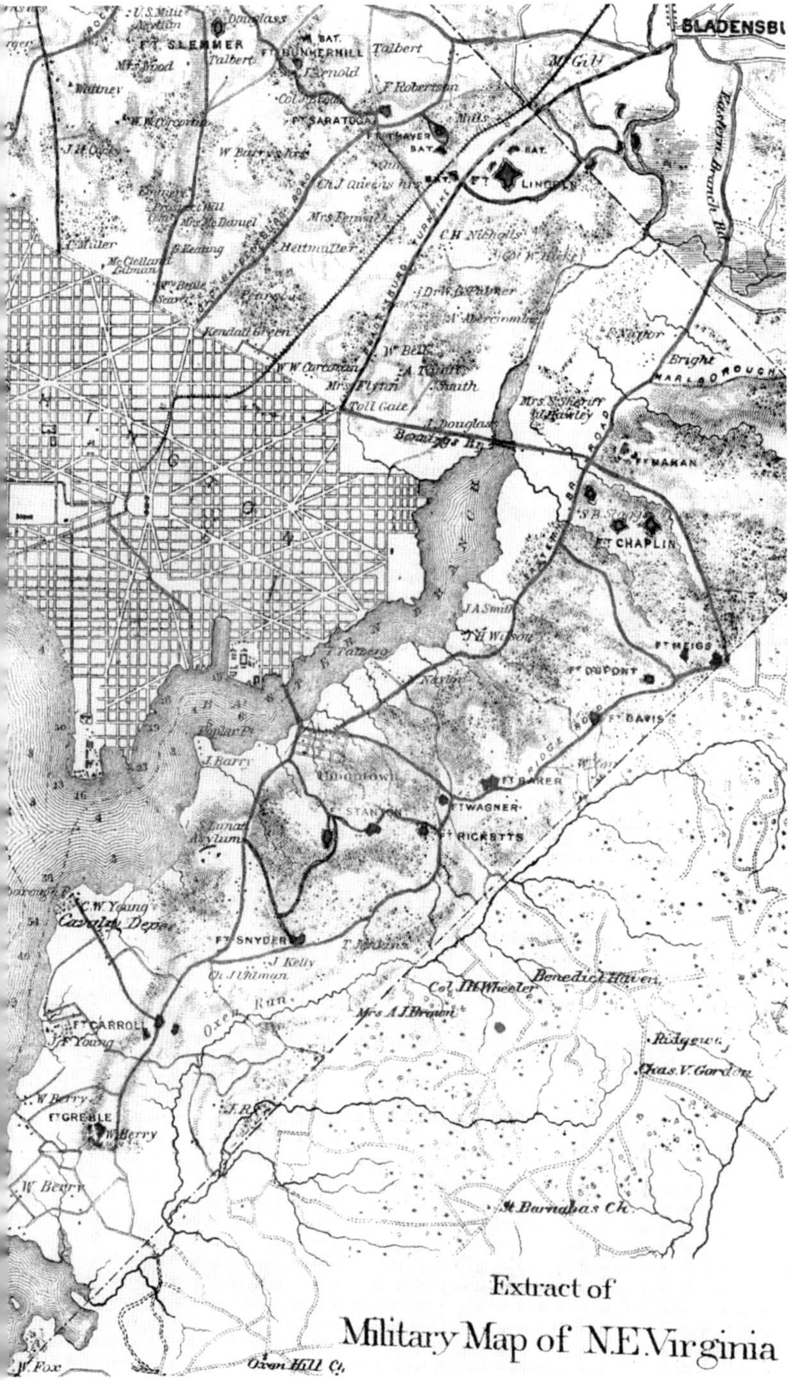

A map of Washington in 1865. *Courtesy of the Library of Congress, Washington, D.C.*

board of twelve managers oversaw the National Asylum. Eventually, there were eleven national homes. Richardson said. "In 1873, they [the board] renamed it the National Home for Disabled Volunteer Soldiers because the word asylum was starting to have negative connotations."[247]

A letter regarding care of soldiers from Cornelia Hancock is quite illustrative:

> *My dear Sister, I shall depict our wants in true but ardent words, hoping to affect you to some action. Here are gathered the sick from the contraband camps in the northern part of Washington. If I were to describe this hospital it would not be believed. North of Washington, in an open, muddy mire, are gathered all the colored people who have been made free by the progress of our Army. Sickness is inevitable, and to meet it these rude hospitals, only rough wooden barracks, are in use—a place where there is so much to be done you need not remain idle. We average here one birth per day, and have no baby clothes except as we wrap them up in an old piece of muslin, that even being scarce. This hospital is the reservoir for all cripples, diseased, aged, wounded, infirm, from whatsoever cause; all accidents happening to colored people in all employs around Washington are brought here. It is not uncommon for a colored driver to be pounded nearly to death by some of the white soldiers. A woman was brought here with three children by her side; said she had been on the road for some time; a more forlorn, worn out looking creature I never beheld. Her four eldest children are still in Slavery, her husband is dead. November 5, 1863.*[248]

In October 1863, Cornelia Hancock traveled to Washington in order to care for freed slaves. She was appalled by the conditions that individuals were living in, writing about smallpox, poor public health and rats:

> *A contraband is a breathing human being capable of being developed, if not so now. Let them have the power to appoint officers to have charge of these camps…who will take an interest in the improvement of those under their charge. I feel this to be the duty of every individual to urge upon every senator and congressman that this step be taken. But meanwhile as we stand at present, our needs are very pressing.*[249]

5
African American Healthcare Providers in D.C. after the Civil War

The experiences of African American physicians, nurses and healthcare workers after the war varied greatly.[250] Some went on to greatness in academia and private practice, and others rejected the medical profession entirely. This chapter will not take an exhaustive look at all providers but will focus on certain surgeons, nurses and others to give an overview of their experiences.

Medical Societies

Several African American physicians, including Alexander Augusta, attempted to become members of white established societies after the war, such as the American Medical Association (AMA). When denied admittance into organizations such as the AMA, they began their own organizations. Augusta founded what would become the National Medical Association, which remains in existence today. The achievements in medicine that these great African American healthcare providers attained paved the way for many others after them to enroll in medical school and go on to achieve their own successes in the medical arena.[251]

For example, after the Civil War, Augusta and Purvis were proposed and then rejected for membership in the Medical Society of the District of Columbia, an affiliate of the American Medical Association. Senator

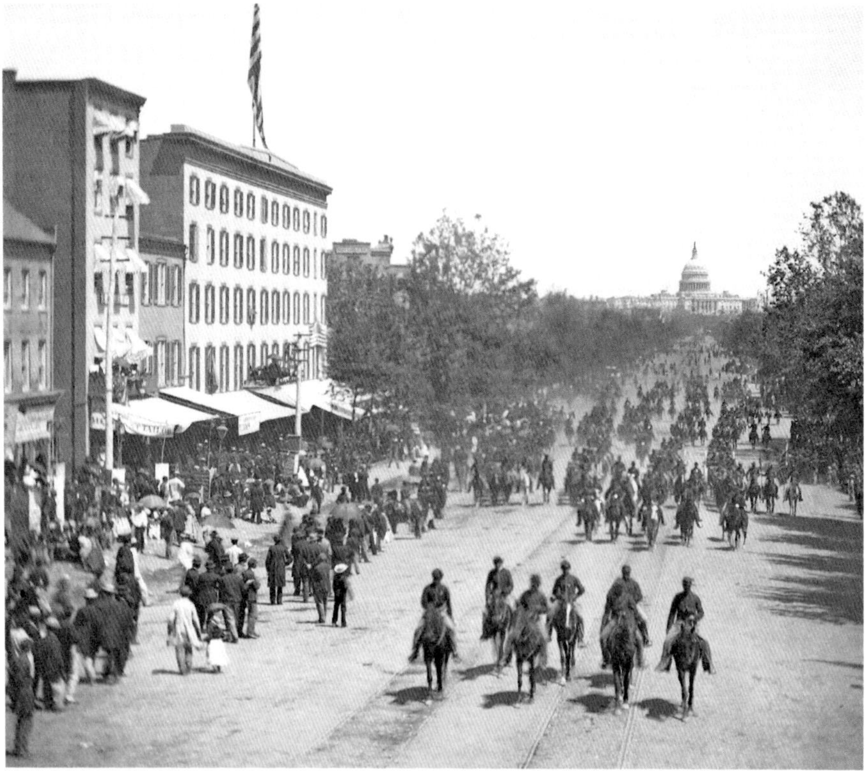

The Grand Review in Washington, D.C., May 1865. *Courtesy of the Library of Congress, Washington, D.C.*

Charles Sumner of Massachusetts introduced a bill in the United States Senate to repeal the charter of the Medical Society of the District of Columbia because it discriminated against practitioners "solely on account of color." The bill was unsuccessful, and the fight continued. On January 15, 1870, African Americans formed the National Medical Society of the District of Columbia and accepted whites into membership.[252]

In 1870, three regularly educated, licensed black physicians—Augusta, Purvis and Alpheus W. Tucker—sought recognition as delegates at the AMA's 1870 meeting in Washington, D.C. Service as a delegate was the primary route to AMA membership. At the 1870 meeting, various physicians lodged ethics complaints against three societies. Each had strong racial implications. The first was a complaint by the National Medical Society, the Medical Society of the District of Columbia and the Massachusetts Medical Society. The all-white Medical Society of the District of Columbia challenged the seating of all members of the National Medical Society, claiming that it "was formed in contempt of" and had "attempted, through legislative influence, to break down" the Medical Society of the District of Columbia by petitioning Congress to address racial discrimination within the society. The National Medical Society, in turn, charged the Medical Society of the District of Columbia with licensing "irregular" practitioners. Lastly, dissident Massachusetts physicians charged their own state society with accepting "irregulars" into membership. Irregulars, such as Thomsonians and homeopaths, were held to practice "an exclusive dogma to the rejection of the accumulated experience of the profession," an important issue for the AMA, since its members competed with irregulars and considered them to be unscientific.

All three cases were referred to the AMA's committee on ethics. That committee found the charge regarding the Medical Society of the District of Columbia's granting licenses to irregulars was "not of a nature to require the action of the [AMA]" and excluded the all-white delegation. The committee also urged recognition of the all-white Massachusetts Medical Society delegation, even though the charge that they accepted irregulars as members was "fully proved" and "plainly in violation of the Code of Ethics." With respect to the integrated National Medical Society, however, following protracted deliberation, the committee remained divided—2 to 3. The minority wanted to recognize the National Medical Society members. The majority urged excluding them. When the issue was put to a roll call vote—in which the thirty-six delegates from the Medical Society of the District of Columbia, but not the National Medical Society, were allowed to vote—the minority report was tabled, 114 to 82, and the majority report was adopted, resulting in the exclusion of National Medical Society members from the AMA.

Following the vote, two Massachusetts delegates, Horatio R. Storer and John L. Sullivan, explicitly raised the issue of race. Amid "a storm of hisses" countered by "Go on! Go on!" Sullivan proposed that the AMA adopt a policy that "no distinction of race or color shall exclude from the Association persons claiming admission and duly accredited thereto." The convention postponed action on this so that Davis could further clarify the ethics committee's reasoning. Davis reiterated that the National Medical Society "used unfair and dishonorable means to procure the destruction" of the Medical Society of the District of Columbia and added that some members of the National Medical Society were not licensed to practice medicine in Washington, D.C. Nothing was said of the many AMA delegates who were not licensed in D.C. or that licenses were issued by the all-white Medical Society of the District of Columbia.

Sullivan's proposal was then tabled. Storer, who had supported admission of National Medical Society members, then proposed a resolution stating that Davis had "distinctly stated and proved that the consideration of race and color has had nothing whatsoever to do with the decision." This motion passed.

The AMA, thus, declined to embrace a policy of nondiscrimination and excluded all members of the integrated National Medical Society. It excluded them by selectively enforcing membership standards, allowing leniency to two all-white delegations that had breached scientific credentialing standards while sanctioning an integrated society, and, immediately thereafter, officially absolving itself of the charge of racism. The AMA must have recognized that its decision had the effect of racial discrimination. In fact, some physicians found it condemnable. Indeed one white commentator, reflecting on the decision, wrote, "I doubt whether, in the last fifty years, a national scientific body has convened anywhere that would have excluded a competent scientist on the ground of color." The AMA, he noted, had put up "new barriers to entrance" and, in doing so, "unharnessed itself from its code of ethics."[253]

Families

Purvis married twice, once to a woman by the name of Ann Hathaway. Purvis's wife Ann, whom he married in April 13, 1871, was white. This was probably fairly difficult for both of them, given the times in which they lived. They had two children—Alice, who became a doctor, and Robert, who became a dentist.[254] After the death of Purvis's first wife, Ann, he married Jenny C. Butman in 1901.

Alpheus Tucker married Martha Ellen Wood on January 26, 1867. They had one child named Sarah Estella. The family lived in Washington, D.C., until 1878, when they moved to Detroit, where Tucker was born. Tucker died in January 1880, and his wife and child moved back to Washington, D.C., to live with his wife's parents. Tucker's wife died on March 14, 1921.

Dr. Creed would go back to Connecticut after the Civil War and marry Drucilla Wright. They had four children. He then married Mary Paul and had six children with her.

Henry Turner married four times. He was married the longest to Eliza Peacher with whom he had fourteen children. She died in 1889, and he then married Martha Elizabeth DeWitt, Harriet Wayman and Laura Pearl Lemon.[255] Willis Revels's brother Hiram was the first African American to be seated in the United States Senate, serving in D.C. from February 1870 to March 1871.

CAREERS

After his time in the Civil War, Charles Purvis taught medicine for many years at the predominately white Howard University. Due to the university's budget constraints, Purvis worked unpaid from 1873 to 1907 and supported himself through his medical practice. In 1873, Purvis wrote to General Oliver Otis Howard, the university president, stating: "While I regret the university will not be able to pay me for my services, I feel the importance of every effort being made to carry forward the institution and to make it a success."[256] Purvis also lobbied Congress to appropriate $600,000 to the school for a new building to house the Freedmen's Hospital.

Between 1869 and 1873, Purvis lectured on many topics, including materia medica, or the science of drugs to treat illnesses; therapeutics; botany; and medical jurisprudence. He was also a professor of obstetrics, gynecology and diseases of women and pediatrics from 1873 to 1889. The board of trustees conferred an honorary degree on Purvis in 1871. From 1883 to 1893, he was chief surgeon at Freedmen's Hospital.

Author John Muller tells the story of how Charles Purvis came to the defense of Frederick Douglass in 1875 after Douglass gave a speech that was somewhat controversial:

> *Douglass had been misunderstood, disputed the physician at Freedmen's Hospital, Charles B. Purvis, a member of a small fraternity of black surgeons commissioned by the U.S. Army during the civil War. "I think he refers more to Washington as it was prior to the war than it is today." Purvis said he knew of the daily pressure and burden, as he felt it "in* [his] *profession, being denied access to institutions established solely for the purpose of discussing medical subjects, simply on account of color, meeting rebuffs from the people."*[257]

In 1904, Purvis became licensed to practice medicine in Massachusetts and was accepted into the Massachusetts Medical Society. On July 2, 1881, Purvis's life would change with the assassination of President James A. Garfield. Leaving for vacation that day by train from the Baltimore and Potomac Railroad Station, Garfield was shot by Charles Guiteau and died eleven weeks later on September 19, 1881. He was accompanied by his two sons, as well as Secretary of State Blaine and Secretary of War Robert Todd Lincoln.[258] He had no security detail. Purvis was one of the surgeons who treated Garfield. When Garfield asked him what his chance for survival was, he uttered the fateful words, "One chance in one hundred." Purvis would go on to be the head of Freedmen's Hospital from 1883 to 1893.

Purvis relocated to Boston, Massachusetts, in 1905 and resigned his teaching position at Howard University in 1907. He was elected to the board of directors at Howard University in 1908 and then resigned this post in 1926. Purvis died in Los Angeles, California, in 1929.[259]

Alexander Augusta married Mary O. Burgoin in January 1847. She would be with him after the war, and they made a life for themselves in Washington, D.C. In 1865 and 1866, Augusta was assigned to the Department of the South and, in 1865, was promoted to lieutenant colonel in the United States Volunteers. He was the first African American to hold that rank. Augusta was mustered out of service on October 13, 1866. He was in charge of the Lincoln Hospital in Savannah, Georgia, until 1868, when he started his own practice in Washington, D.C. He also served at the Smallpox Hospital and Freedmen's Hospital, both in D.C. In 1868, Augusta was added to the medical department of Howard University, making him the first African American to be offered a teaching position at a medical school in the country. As was mentioned before, due to financial constraints, the school was unable to pay its faculty, and many resigned. Augusta remained, however, and continued on faculty until September 1877, when he reentered private practice.

On September 21, 1868, when Augusta was appointed to the five-member medical faculty as a demonstrator of anatomy, he was the first African American to hold a faculty position at a medical school in the United States. "In 1877, after the medical faculty recommended to the trustees that Augusta switch positions with Dr. Daniel Lamb and become chair of materia medica rather than anatomy, Augusta resigned and returned to private practice."[260]

John H. Rapier Jr., frustrated by the racial climate in the United States, pursued professional opportunities in the Caribbean. However, he returned to the United States to complete a medical degree and became one of the first acting assistant surgeons at the Freedmen's Hospital.

Cortlandt Van Rensselaer Creed went on to practice in Connecticut for most of his career and for a short amount of time in Brooklyn, New York. He was consulted on President Garfield's assassination in 1881.

After the Civil War ended, Sojourner Truth continued working to help the newly freed slaves through the Freedmen's Relief Association. In 1867, she moved from Harmonia to Battle Creek. In 1870, she began campaigning for the federal government to provide former slaves with land in the new West. This was a campaign that she championed for many years. She was ill through the 1870s but continued to champion the rights of former slaves. In 1879, she would see former slaves begin to migrate

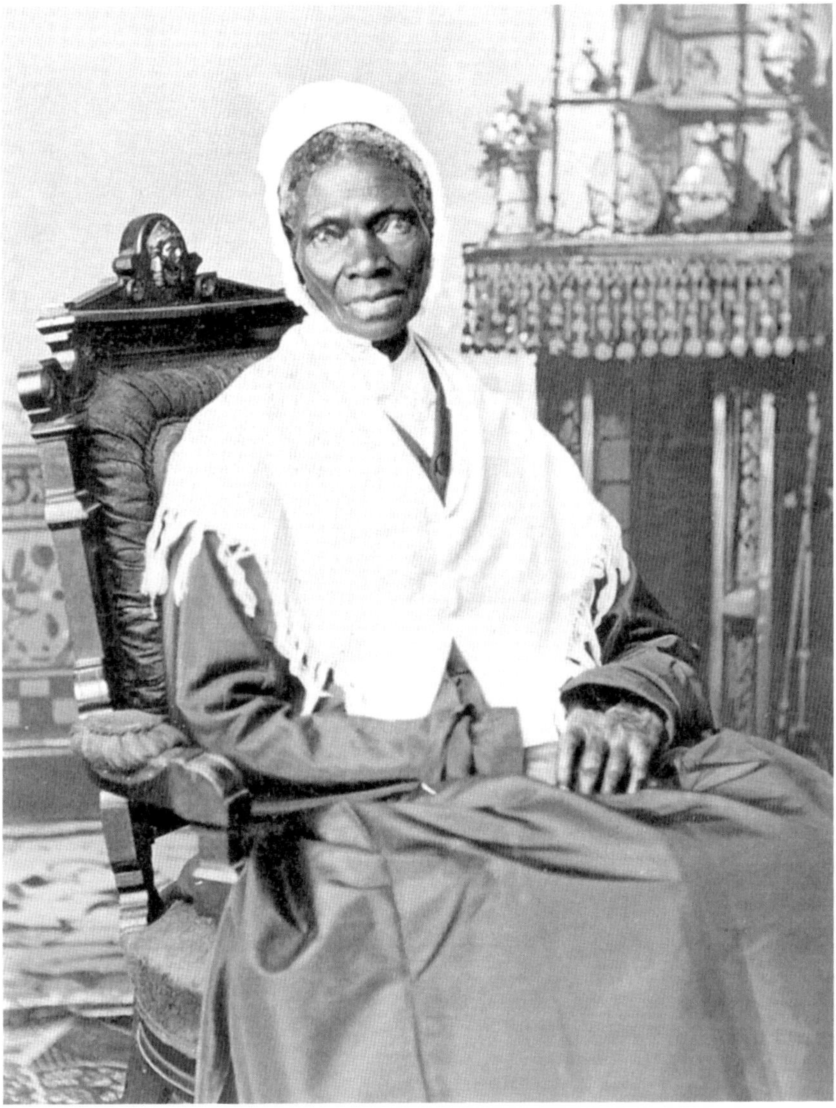

Sojourner Truth. *Courtesy of the National Portrait Gallery, Smithsonian Institution.*

north and west and spent time getting support for the migrants as they began to build lives for themselves. She would take some appearances in the 1880s but became very ill due to ulcers on her legs. She had skin grafts to treat the ulcers but returned home and died November 26, 1883, at the age of eighty-six.

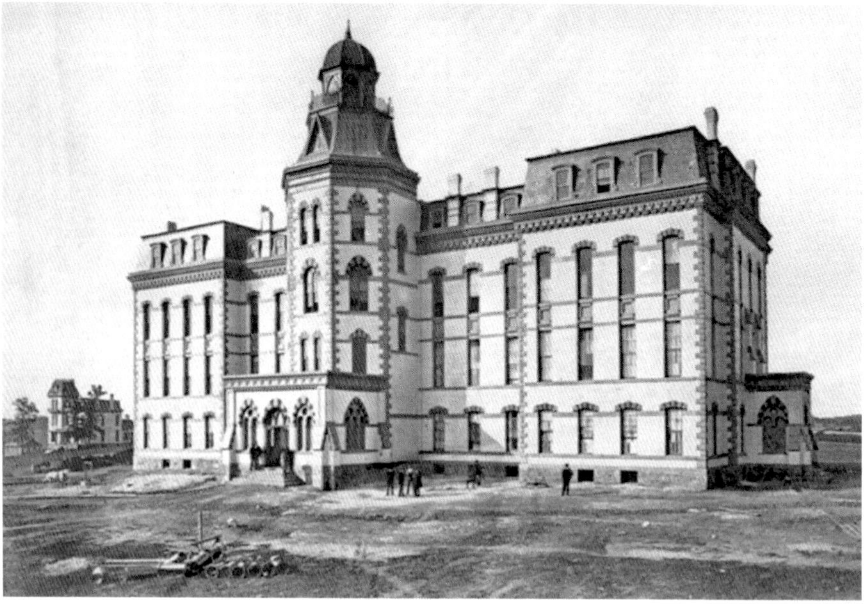

Howard University's Old Main Building in the 1860s. *Courtesy of the Howard University Archives.*

For Henry Turner, there were many decisions to make postwar—what to do with the rest of his life, both with respect to his career and his personal life, and how to continue the important work that had started during the war. Immediately after the war, Turner returned to Washington and spent time with Bishop Daniel Payne. He wished to organize a mission to the South to work with the newly freed slaves. He approached the mission board of the AME Church. However, they were in as dire financial straits, as most others during this time period.

Alpheus Tucker was from Michigan and graduated from the Iowa College of Physicians and Surgeons in 1865. He was part of the Contraband Hospital in Washington, D.C., and remained in Washington after the war. Along with Dr. Augusta and Charles Purvis, Tucker applied for and was denied admittance to membership in the District of Columbia's medical society in 1869.[261]

Ever the champion of the rights of African Americans, after being repeatedly denied admittance to various white medical societies, in 1884 Augusta became one of the founding members of the Medico-Chirurgical Society, the first African American medical society in the United States.[262]

Augusta died on December 21, 1890, at age sixty-five. He was buried in section one of Arlington National Cemetery with full military honors.[263] Augusta is primarily remembered today for being the first African American surgeon in the Union army and the first African American officer-rank soldier to be buried at Arlington Cemetery.

The greatness of Dr. Augusta cannot be understated. In addition to the barriers that he brought down in the medical arena, he was a civil rights leader for his time, championing the rights of the oppressed, as well as a trailblazer in various businesses with his wife before the Civil War. This he did while constantly battling bigotry and ignorance and fighting to be able to excel in his profession.

Before the Civil War, Joseph Dennis Harris, from Virginia wrote a book supporting colonization for African Americans and went to Haiti to promote that cause. He later decided on medicine as a career and, after one year at the Medical Department of Western Reserve College (now Western Reserve University), he served in Virginia where he remained after the war. In 1869, Harris was a candidate for lieutenant governor of Virginia but did not win the election. His date of death is not known.

Pensions and Postwar Military Recognition

On February 18, 1891, Anderson Abbott wrote a letter to the secretary of war requesting an increase in his rank from his time serving in the Civil War. That his mentor, Alexander Augusta, had died the year before might have influenced Powell's decision to write such a letter.

> *Dear Sir: I am one of those who left Canada during the late Civil War to assist the government of the United States in suppressing the rebellion in the south. My services were accepted in 1863, and I served as Act. Asst. Surgeon until the close of the war. I endeavoured to discharge the duties assigned me to the best of my ability as may be seen by examining the enclosed copies of testimonials the originals of which I have in my possession. I was placed on duty in the hospital in Washington DC which was there under the charge of the late surgeon Augusta, US Vols. In a short time I was promoted to the position of surgeon in charge and*

> *remained in charge of hospitals until the close of the war. As an evidence that I was held in some esteem during my sojourn in Washington allow me to mention that after the death of Mr. Lincoln, Mrs. Lincoln sent me, as a memento, the plaid shawl which he wore on his way to the first of many* [events] *and which is alleged, formed part of a disguise which he wore on that occasion. I hope it will not be deemed presumption on my part in asking the government to grant me an honorary or brevet rank in the United States military service, in recognition of the services I rendered. I am now an old man, and as I grow older I appreciate more highly the part (though humble) that in those…times and which resulted in the emancipation of my race in the United States. If it is in the power of the government to grant my request I pray that my case may receive a favourable consideration. It is my intention to visit Washington the latter part of March and if a personal interview is desirable I would be very glad if you would intimate the same and I shall be very happy to call upon you.*[264]

William Powell would spend the rest of his life petitioning for his pension, which the government denied due to lack of evidence of the nature and severity of his disability and the fact that he was not commissioned but rather contracted with the army to perform his duties. A catch-twenty-two about the pension system is that it was more challenging for African Americans to prove their medical disabilities were war related.[265] Powell died in 1915 in England, never having received his pension, confined to a home for the aged and infirmed.[266]

With a special act of Congress, Civil War nurses received pensions thirty years after the end of the war. Harriet Tubman also received a special pension due to her service, but Susie King Taylor did not, in part because she was not classified as a nurse. On September 16, 1866, Taylor's first husband died, and Taylor, now with a baby, returned to Savannah and opened a school for students to attend at night and also taught adults. Another school opened and put her school out of business again, so Taylor was forced to leave her baby with her mother and go to work for a family.[267] Taylor would work for various other families until she met and then married Russell Taylor in 1879. Taylor also remained devoted to others, organizing the Women's Relief Corps, auxiliary to the Grand Army of the Republic, and in 1896, she assisted in the census to secure a complete roster of the Union veterans living in Massachusetts. This she did with Lizzie L. Johnson, widow of a soldier of the Fifty-fourth Massachusetts.

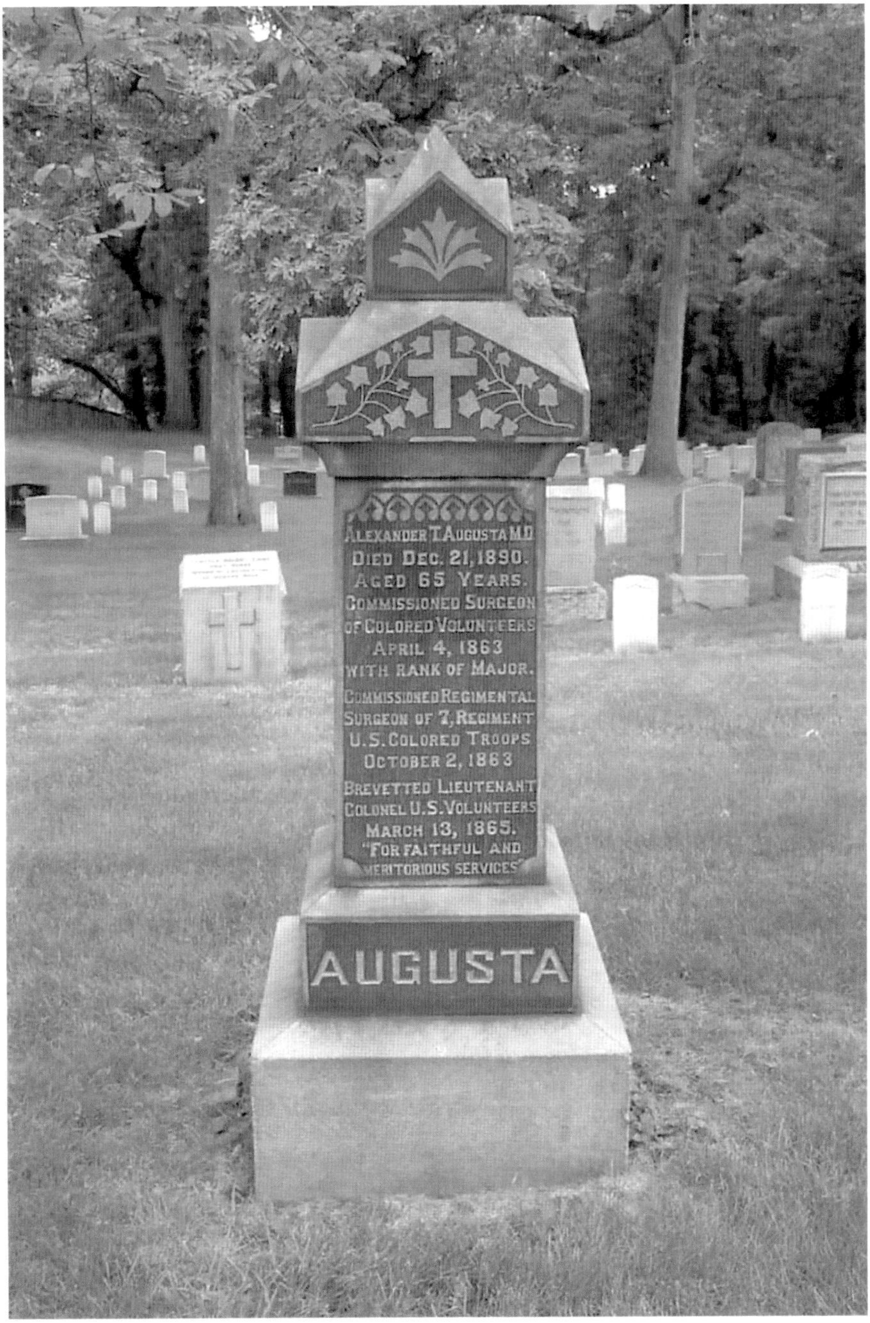
ALEXANDER T. AUGUSTA M.D
DIED DEC. 21, 1890.
AGED 65 YEARS.
COMMISSIONED SURGEON
OF COLORED VOLUNTEERS
APRIL 4, 1863
WITH RANK OF MAJOR.
COMMISSIONED REGIMENTAL
SURGEON OF 7, REGIMENT
U.S. COLORED TROOPS
OCTOBER 2, 1863
BREVETTED LIEUTENANT
COLONEL U.S. VOLUNTEERS
MARCH 13, 1865.
"FOR FAITHFUL AND
MERITORIOUS SERVICES"
AUGUSTA

The headstone of Dr. Alexander Augusta at Arlington Cemetery. *Courtesy of M.R. Patterson.*

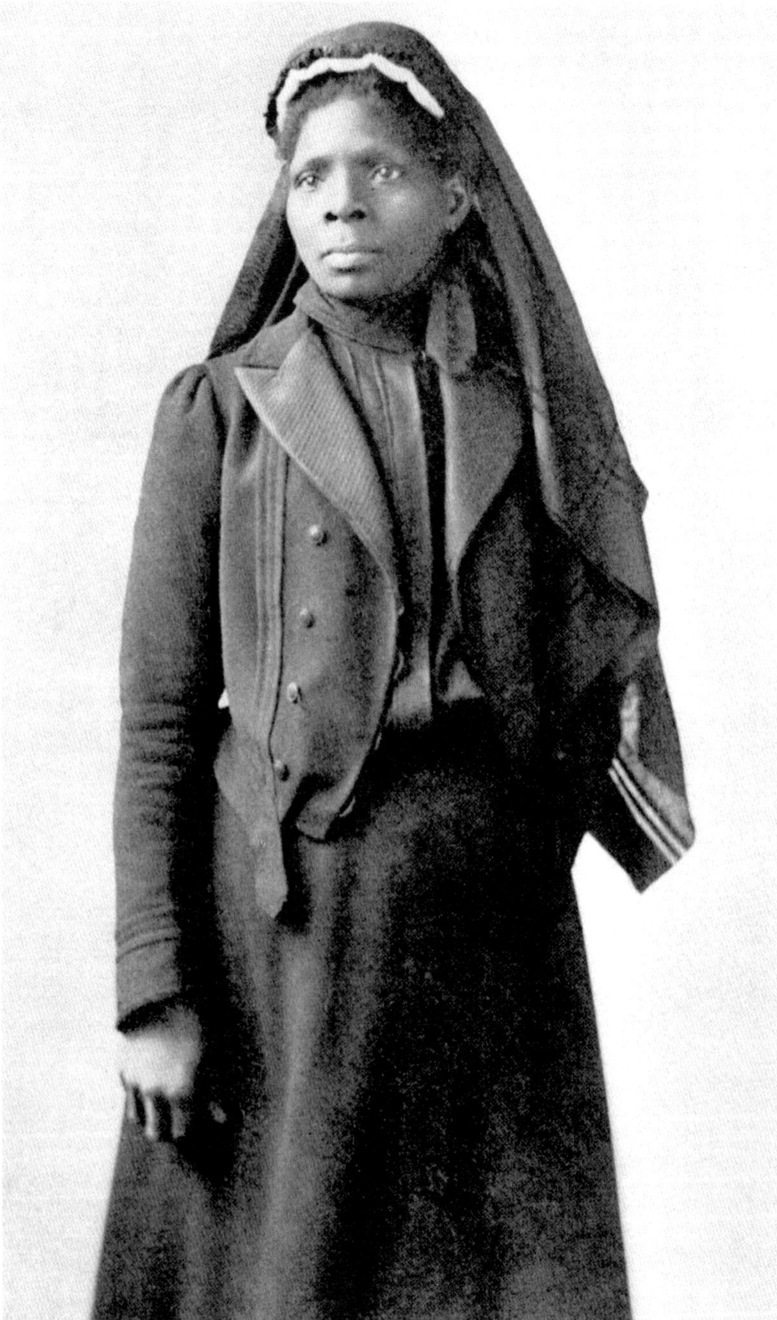

Susie King Taylor. *Courtesy of the National Gallery of Art.*

Pension records are a rich source of information regarding individuals due to the amount of detail that had to be supplied to support the pension application. Ann Stokes first applied for a pension in 1889 based on her husband's service. Stokes married her husband on December 24, 1866. John West and Alfred Ferguson of the USS *Red Rover* witnessed the marriage. There is no information on the disposition of the pension application, but Stokes was already remarried, which would have prevented her from getting the pension from Gilbert Stokes.

On July 25, 1890, Ann Stokes applied for an invalid pension under the Act of June 27, 1890. She was sixty years old and living in Belknap, Johnson County, Illinois, and her case was taken under review. Her pension application confirmed that Stokes was a nurse in the navy from January 1, 1863, to October 25, 1864. She was given an exam in keeping with the pension application. She was described as "quite large," had given birth to one child and "moved about slowly." According to the Act of June 27, 1890, regarding pensions: "All persons who served ninety days or more in the military or naval service of the United States during the late war of the rebellion, and who had been honorably discharged there from, shall upon making due proof be placed upon the list of invalid pensioners of the United States."[268] "Persons" is not described as being a man or a woman. She was found, based on her pension exam, to be disabled in keeping with the pension regulations. According to the law division: "I cannot find any authority of law for refusing to pension this woman simply because she served as a nurse, as the law under which she seeks pension does not specify in what capacity the persons eligible thereunder shall have served, nor is the question of sex mentioned in the law." Stokes did in fact receive her pension of twelve dollars per month as of July 1890.[269]

Lucy Berrington died in the hospital that she worked at in New Bern, and there was no pension filed for her.[270]

As stated earlier, Harriet Tubman was born in 1820 (approximately) in Dorchester, Maryland. She married John Tubman in 1844 and escaped slavery to Philadelphia, Pennsylvania, in 1849. Tubman started the famed Underground Railroad in 1850 and, in 1857, purchased a home in Auburn, New York, for her parents. She served as a Civil War nurse and scout and, after the war, returned home to Auburn, New York. In 1867, Tubman's first husband, John Tubman, died and she later married Nelson Davis. In 1890, Tubman applied for a Civil War Veteran's pension, and in 1900, she was granted a widow's pension of twenty dollars per month.

Newspapers were an additional way to recognize African American Civil War veterans. They flourished in postwar Washington, D.C. The *Washington Afro-American Newspaper* was founded in 1892 by Sergeant John H. Murphy, a veteran of the war.[271] The *Washington Bee* was founded in 1882. It was edited by William Chase, an African American lawyer and journalist.[272]

At the second session of the 107th Congress, May 15, 2000, (legislative day, May 9, 2002), Senator Hillary Clinton of New York, due in no small measure to a group of students from the Albany Free School who visited the senator and had studied the life of Tubman, submitted the following resolution:

> *Expressing the sense of Congress that Harriet Tubman should have been paid a pension for her service as a nurse and scout in the United States Army during the Civil War.*
>
> *Whereas during the Civil War Harriet Tubman reported to General David Hunter at Hilton Head, South Carolina, with a letter from Governor John Andrews of Massachusetts allowing her to serve in the Union Army;*
>
> *Whereas Harriet Tubman served at Hilton Head as a nurse, scout, spy, and cook;*
>
> *Whereas in the spring of 1865, Harriet Tubman worked at the Freedmen's hospital in Fortress Monroe, Virginia;*
>
> *Whereas Harriet Tubman's last husband, Nelson Davis, served in the United States Colored infantry under Captain James S. Thompson, beginning on September 25, 1863, and was discharged on November 10, 1865;*
>
> *Whereas Harriet Tubman received a pension as the spouse of a deceased veteran;*
>
> *Whereas Harriet Tubman requested a pension for her own service in the Union Army during the Civil War, but never received one;*
>
> *Whereas a bill that passed the House of Representatives in 1897 during the 55th Congress (H.R. 4982) would have required that Harriet Tubman be placed on the pension roll of the United States for her service as a nurse in the United States Army and paid a pension at the rate of $25 each month;*
>
> *Whereas some females who served in the military during the Civil War received a pension for their service, including Sarah Emma Edmonds Seelye and Alberta Cashier, each of whom posed as a male; and*
>
> *Whereas Harriet Tubman died of pneumonia on March 10, 1913, and was buried at Fort Hill Cemetery in Auburn, New York, with military honors; Now, therefore, be it Resolved by the Senate (the House of Representatives concurring), That—*

> *(1) Congress recognize that Harriet Tubman served as a nurse and scout in the United States Army during the Civil War; and (2) It is the sense of Congress that Harriet Tubman should have been paid a pension at the rate of $25 each month for her service in the United States Army.*[273]

Howard University recognized its star medical school faculty on June 27, 1871, when it awarded honorary degrees to Augusta, Purvis and Robert Reyburn. Augusta also received an honorary degree of medicinal doctor on June 30, 1896. In honor of the noted surgeon and educator, in 1913 doctors Simeon L. Carson, B. Price Hurst, Peter M. Murray and E.A. Robinson formed the Alexander T. Augusta Medical Reading Club.

As stated earlier, Augusta died on December 21, 1890, at age sixty-five, and he was buried in section one of Arlington National Cemetery with full military honors. Augusta was the first African American surgeon in the Union army and the first African American officer-rank soldier to be buried at Arlington Cemetery. But we remember him not only for those accomplishments, as stunning as they were for an African American banned from United States medical schools, but also for the whole fertile creative life that he led:

> *Commissioned surgeon of colored volunteers, April 4, 1863, with the rank of Major. Commissioned regimental surgeon of the 7th Regiment of US. Colored Troops, October 2, 1863. Brevet Lieutenant Colonel of Volunteers, March 13, 1865, for faithful and meritorious services-mustered out October 13, 1866.*[274]

EPILOGUE

The history of medical care of African American soldiers during the Civil War is one that often is tangentially included and then lost within the history of overall medical care during the war. While many African American soldiers and healthcare workers had to face great adversity and prejudice, the positives for many African Americans to represent their country and serve in such an important endeavor made facing such difficulties worthwhile.

Several things can be concluded. First, African Americans entered the wartime effort, both as soldiers and healthcare providers, uniquely. The definitive work "A Peculiar Population: The Nutrition, Health, and Mortality of American Slaves from Childhood to Maturity" aptly demonstrates this point. In the article, Steckel concludes that slave children were poorly fed and suffered from nutritional deficiencies but that slaves were able to adapt and have growth pattern recovery that was unique in comparison to other similarly situated groups. It speaks to a level of resiliency among the slaves that is commendable.[275] It is data such as this that in retrospect gives a different view of healthcare of African American soldiers during the war and how these soldiers entered the war from a healthcare perspective.

Second, African American healthcare providers of all levels had an arduous time in terms of being able to utilize their talents to serve their country. This is clear from the lack of ties many healthcare providers had to D.C. at the beginning of the war. From surgeons to nurses to stewards, being able to use their skill and ability to heal others was no easy task for African American healthcare workers. Dr. Anderson Abbott, an African Canadian, is but one example of the many surgeons who had to plead with the government to utilize them in their capacity as doctors and nurses during the war. We have heard his words earlier in this book: "I beg most respectfully to apply for a situation as medical Cadet in the army."[276] They ring no less true at the conclusion. Half the battle for most African Americans was in proving to their own government that they would be a positive force in the war.

Third, healthcare generally for all of the sick and wounded during the war was deplorable because of the lack of knowledge regarding infections, anesthesia, how diseases spread and hygiene. Bollet, in his article "An Analysis of the Medical Problems of the Civil War," speaks about these diseases, from diarrhea and dysentery to scurvy, as well as the diet, mainly of hardtack, that soldiers had to endure. Even night blindness is attributable to poor nutrition:

> *Scurvy first became a notable problem during McClellan's peninsular campaign during the spring and summer of 1862. McClellan's medical staff was surprised, since they thought men were eating the desiccated vegetables…Another classic nutritional deficiency syndrome which affects Civil War troops was night blindness…Physicians considered it a bizarre form of malingering, since affected men had to be led by the hand at night, but could not go into battle next morning.*[277]

This should not be confused with the care that the vast majority of healthcare workers, both African American and white, gave to their patients and their craft. The medical aftermath of the Civil War led to great gains in the public health arena with respect to everything from anesthesia to wound infection control and abdominal surgery. Surgeons in the war worked with the tools that they had at the time, and their efforts were not in vain.

Fourth, while some white surgeons and nurses carried with them certain biases with respect to their patients, the war would assist in helping these healers have a different view of African American patients—thanks to both the courage and the valor of the African American soldiers who took part in the war effort. Anderson Abbott tells the story of Dr. Cronyn, president of the examining board for the Army Medical Department, examining Abbott's mentor, Alexander Augusta, for services as a surgeon in the Civil War. After Augusta passed the examination, Surgeon General Hammond asked how Cronyn let Augusta pass to which Cronyn admitted that Augusta knew more than he did "and I could not help myself."[278] This was especially true after the war, when surgeons such as Augusta made Washington, D.C., their home and changed the face of medicine not only in D.C. but also in the country as a whole.

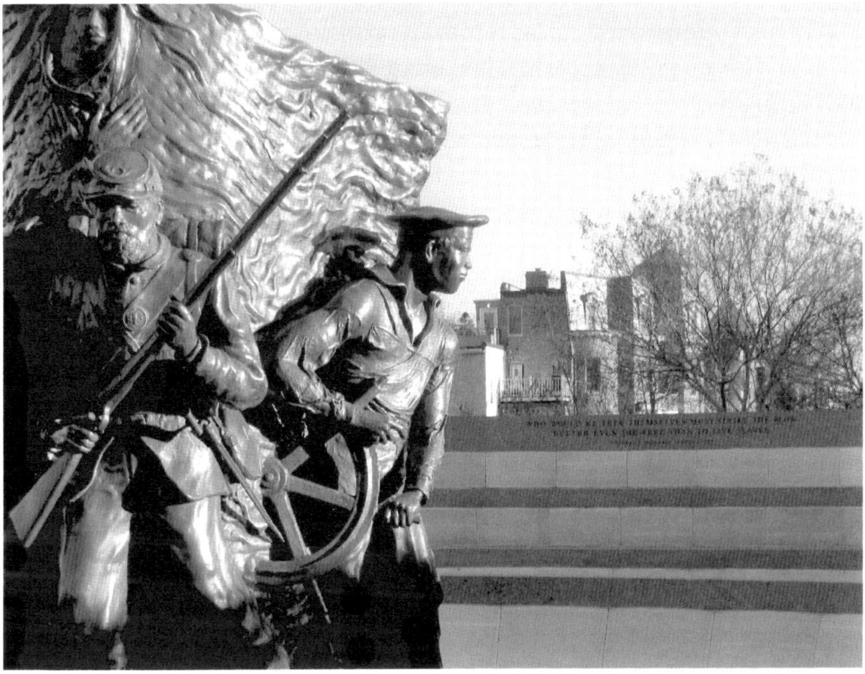

An African American Civil War museum sculpture. *Courtesy of the Library of Congress, Washington, D.C.*

Fifth, as stated earlier, African American physicians had a very difficult time getting into the war as healers to begin with but once they were able to participate, they did so with the same courage that soldiers and others in the army served. Because many African Americans had difficulty even obtaining healthcare training that would qualify them to serve in the army, the fact that they were able to serve and do so most admirably is a credit to them and their struggle to give back to their country and the sick and wounded of the war.

Sixth, the work that African American nurses and other healers did in the armed services led in no small measure to the success of the war. Much like the surgeons, African American nurses had to struggle in order to serve their country and give back. Likewise, healers such as chaplains and stewards would face racial discrimination and prejudice but valiantly fought in the face of such odds.

Seventh, there were many lessons that the armed services took away from the work of African American healers. The pension system and how African Americans were treated in that system is one example. In his article "Prejudice and Policy," Sven E. Wilson notes: "the pension assistance received by black veterans was a financial lifeline to them as well as to their families and communities. But in this, as with so many other matters, black veterans were not given their fair share."[279] Through perseverance and fighting on the part of several African American veterans of the war effort including individuals such as Sojourner Truth, African Americans would begin to get their due with respect to equal pension rights, as they received what they were owed with respect to equal pay in the war. This would be a lesson that the armed services would incorporate into its culture and would serve well in future wars and conflicts.

Finally, the contributions that African American healers gave to this country after the war are incalculable. From continuing to heal others to beginning medical associations and nursing programs and teaching in esteemed schools throughout the country, the African American healers of the war would continue to contribute to this country and partner with others to make this the true United States of America.

NOTES

CHAPTER 1

1. Hunter, "For Freed Blacks in the Civil War."
2. Schroeder-Lein, *Encyclopedia of Civil War Medicine*, 330.
3. Emancipation Day, "Ending Slavery in the District of Columbia." "Though the Compensated Emancipation Act was an important legal and symbolic victory it was part of a larger struggle over the meaning and practice of freedom and citizenship."
4. Ibid.
5. Newmark, "Contraband Hospital."
6. Hunter, "For Freed Blacks in the Civil War."
7. Ibid.
8. Abdy, "Journal of a Residence and Tour in the United States."
9. United States Census Bureau. "Census of Population and Housing."
10. Ibid.
11. Ibid.
12. Ibid.
13. Lowe, "Nineteenth Century Review of Mental Healthcare for African Americans."
14. Ibid.
15. Ibid.
16. Gates, *Classic Slave Narratives*, 74.
17. Ibid., 75.
18. Ibid.
19. Margo and Steckel, "Heights of American Slaves," 517.

20. Steckel, "Peculiar Population," 726.
21. Ibid.
22. Margo and Steckel, "Heights of American Slaves," 517.
23. Steckel, "Peculiar Population," 732–33.
24. Ibid.
25. Whitman, *Leaves of Grass*, 138–39.
26. Ibid.
27. Savitt, *Four African-American Proprietary Medical Colleges*, 203.
28. African American Registry, "Alexander August: A Pioneering Doctor."
29. Cobb, "Alexander Thomas Augusta, 1825–1890," 327–29.
30. Cobb, "Nathan Frances Mossell," 118–30.
31. Mossell, "Autobiography."
32. Ibid.
33. Butts, "Alexander Thomas Augusta: Physician, Teacher and Human Rights Activist," 106–09.
34. Ibid.
35. Schroeder-Lein, *Encyclopedia of Civil War Medicine*, 329–30.
36. United States Census Bureau. "District of Columbia—Race and Hispanic Origin."
37. Newby, *Anderson Ruffin Abbott*, 60. Newby cites Berlin, Reidy and Rowland, *Freedom: A Documentary History of Emancipation*, 355–56.
38. Redkey, "Henry McNeal Turner: Black Chaplain in the Union Army," 337–38.
39. Emancipation Day, "Ending Slavery in the District of Columbia."
40. Redkey, "Henry McNeal Turner: Black Chaplain in the Union Army," 338.

Chapter 2

41. Adams, *Doctors in Blue*, 113.
42. Ibid., 114. Musket balls made terrible wounds. The musket balls traveled at low velocity, losing shape on impact and often lodging in tissue, carrying skin and clothes, which led to infections.
43. Ibid., 115.
44. Berlin and Fields, *Free at Last*, 477.
45. Bayne-Jones, *Evolution of Preventative Medicine*.
46. MacDonald, *Historical Atlas of the Civil War*, 197.
47. Aptheker, "Negro Casualties in the Civil War," 10–80.
48. Ibid.
49. Byrd and Clayton, *American Health Dilemma*, 385.

50. Glatthaar, *Forged in Battle*, 190–91.
51. Ibid.
52. Ibid., 192.
53. Ibid., 190.
54. Ibid., 187.
55. Ibid., 194.
56. Ibid.
57. Ibid.
58. Oates, *Woman of Valor*, 155.
59. Reid, ed., *Practicing Medicine in a Black Regiment*, 6.
60. Ibid., 52.
61. Ibid., 54.
62. Schwartz, *Woman Doctor's Civil War*, 160, 162. Note in Wilder's book: "In contrast to the descriptions of Brown left by Wilder (and Frank), Esther Hill Hawks described her former teacher as genial and recounted how enjoyable some of the women found his company."
63. Reid, *Practicing Medicine in a Black Regiment*, 54.
64. Ibid., 82.
65. Ibid., 76.
66. Oates, *Woman of Valor*, 155.
67. Alcott, *Hospital Sketches*, 101–02.
68. Zwierzyna, "Nicholas Biddle."
69. Whitman, *Leaves of Grass*, 85–86.
70. Ibid., 116–17
71. Ibid., 138–39
72. Dobak, *Freedom by the Sword*, 34.
73. Ibid., 6.
74. Ibid., 7.
75. Ibid., 10.
76. Ibid.
77. Ibid.
78. Ibid., 12.
79. Sparks, "James Slaughter."
80. Voices of the Civil War, "Christian Fleetwood."
81. Lincoln, "Letter to Horace Greeley."
82. Humphreys, *Intensely Human*, 7.
83. Hunter, "For Freed Blacks in the Civil War."
84. Smith, *Black Soldiers in Blue*, 39.
85. McPherson, *Ordeal by Fire*, 349.

86. Lee, "Socioeconomic Differences in the Health of Black Union Army Soldiers," 434.
87. Dobak, *Freedom by the Sword*, 59.
88. Wilson, *Campfires of Freedom*, 62.
89. Aptheker, "Negro Casualties in the Civil War," 10–80.
90. Ibid.
91. Ibid.
92. Ibid.
93. Steven, "The 1st US Colored Troops at Roosevelt Island."
94. Aptheker, "Negro Casualties in the Civil War," 10–80.
95. Ibid.
96. Ibid.
97. Ibid.
98. Ibid.
99. Ibid. But, of course, the main body of nonenlisted African Americans who served the Union forces worked for army units or for the quartermaster, commissary, medical and engineer services in such occupations as pioneers, laborers, hostlers, teamsters, wagoners, carpenters, masons, laundresses, hospital attendants, fortification, highway and railroad builders, longshoremen and blacksmiths.
100. Ibid.
101. Smith, *Black Soldiers in Blue*, 40.
102. Ibid., 41.
103. Ibid., 62.
104. Ibid., 250.
105. Aptheker, "Negro Casualties in the Civil War," 10–80.
106. Wilson, *Campfires of Freedom*, 63.
107. Aptheker, "Negro Casualties in the Civil War," 10–80.
108. Ibid.
109. Ibid.
110. Humphreys, *Intensely Human*, 7.
111. Ibid.
112. Ibid.
113. Ibid.
114. Glatthaar, *Forged in Battle*, 187.
115. Ibid.
116. Aptheker, "Negro Casualties in the Civil War," 10–80.
117. Garrison, *Civil War Curiosities*, 104. "The soldiers of the 54th Massachusetts Infantry, made famous in the movie *Glory*, refused to accept any pay until

they received pay commensurate with their white counterparts." On page 142 of the book, Garrison states, "As early as August 1862 Secretary of War Edwin M. Stanton had promised African American recruits the same pay as whites ($13 per month, $3 of which constituted a clothing allowance), but in 1863 War Department Solicitor William Whiting ruled that under the Militia Act of July 1862, African Americans of all ranks were to be paid $10 per month with $3 withheld by the government for clothing. [In *The African American in the American Rebellion*] Brown wrote that the men of the Fifty-fourth and Fifty-fifth Massachusetts Volunteers rightly believed that they had been recruited 'under false pretenses,' and the men protested by not accepting wages lower than those of white troops." On page 145, Garrison goes on to state that the men of of the Fifty-fourth were greatly admired "for refusing on principle to accept extra pay offered by Massachusetts to equalize their pay with whites. "Standing by their expressed determination to have justice done them, they quietly performed their duties, only praying earnestly that every friend of theirs at the North would help the Government to see what a blot rests on its fair fame, a betrayal of the trust reposed in them by the colored race. Not until June 1864 did Congress finally equalize pay for African American and white troops."

118. Aptheker, "Negro Casualties in the Civil War," 10–80.
119. Berlin and Fields, *Free at Last*, 450.
120. Ibid., 459.
121. McPherson, *Ordeal by Fire*, 351.
122. Ibid.
123. Humphreys, *Intensely Human*, xii–xvii.
124. Aptheker, "Negro Casualties in the Civil War," 10–80.
125. Ibid.
125. Ibid.
126. Ibid.
127. Ibid.
128. Cunningham, *Doctors in Gray*, 102.
129. Smith, *Black Soldiers in Blue*, 144–45.
130. Humphreys, *Intensely Human*, 7.
131. Ibid.
132. Ibid.
133. Aptheker, "Negro Casualties in the Civil War," 10–80.
134. Ibid.
135. Ibid.

136. Ibid.
137. Ibid.
138. Wilson, *Campfires of Freedom*, 64.
139. Ibid.
140. Schroeder-Lein, *Encyclopedia of Civil War Medicine*, 4.
141. Wilson, *Campfires of Freedom*, 64.
142. Schroeder-Lein, *Encyclopedia of Civil War Medicine*, 3.
143. Ibid.
144. Ibid.
145. Ibid.
146. Ibid.
147. Black, "In the Service of the United States," 317–33.
148. Ibid.
149. Bollet, "Analysis of the Medical Problems of the Civil War," 129.
150. Black, "In the Service of the United States," 317–33.
151. Ibid.
152. Ibid.
153. Sattelmeyer, "Miss Alcott Goes to War," 44.
154. Black, "In the Service of the United States," 317–33.
155. Ibid.
156. Ibid.
157. Ibid.
158. Schroeder-Lein, *Encyclopedia of Civil War Medicine*, 4.
159. Black, "In the Service of the United States," 317–33.
160. Ibid.
161. Ibid.
162. Ibid.
163. Ibid.
164. Ibid.
165. Aptheker, "Negro Casualties in the Civil War," 10–80.
166. Ibid.
167. Ibid.
168. Black, "In the Service of the United," 317–33.
169. Ibid.
170. Schroeder-Lein, *Encyclopedia of Civil War Medicine*, 12.

171. Ibid. In the Confederacy, the Richmond Ambulance Committee, organized in the spring of 1862, seems to have been the first concerted effort to bring order to the transportation chaos on either side. About one hundred prominent Richmond men exempted from military duty volunteered for ambulance service at their own expense. They had thirty-nine ambulances at the Battle of Williamsburg (Virginia) on May 5, 1862, and continued to provide vital aid to the Army of Northern Virginia during the other battles of the Peninsula Campaign.
172. Aptheker, "Negro Casualties in the Civil War," 10–80.
173. Ibid.
174. Wilson, *Campfires of Freedom*, 62.
175. Ibid.
176. Ibid.
177. Aptheker, "Negro Casualties in the Civil War," 10–80.
178. Ibid.
179. Ibid.
180. Ibid.
181. Ibid.
182. Ibid.
183. Wikipedia, "Laura Smith Haviland."
184. Haviland, *Woman's Life-work*, 391–92.
185. Smith, *Black Soldiers in Blue*, 42–43.
186. Aptheker, "Negro Casualties in the Civil War," 10–80.
187. Ibid.
188. Catton and Ketchum, *American Heritage Picture History of the Civil War*, 418–19.
189. Simmons and Turner, *Men of Mark*, 1,007.
190. Catton and Ketchum, *American Heritage Picture History of the Civil War*, 422–23.
191. Aptheker, "Negro Casualties in the Civil War," 10–80.
192. Ibid.
193. Ibid.
194. Ibid.
195. Ibid.
196. Ibid.
197. Ibid.
198. Ibid.
199. Ibid.
200. Ibid.

Chapter 3

201. Harrison, *Washington during the Civil War and Reconstruction*, 34.
202. King, "In Search of Women of African Descent," 303.
203. Benson, "The Role of Chaplains in the Civil War."
204. Cobb, "Alexander Thomas Augusta, 1825–1890," 327. "Apparently the letter had an effect, for Dr. Augusta was placed on detached service examining African American recruits at Benedict and Baltimore, Maryland throughout 1864, and at a recruiting service in the Department of the South thereafter until hostilities were terminated."
205. McPherson, *Negro's Civil War*, 265.
206. Augusta to Captain C.W. Clippington, 265.
207. Ibid.
208. Aptheker, "Negro Casualties in the Civil War ," 10–80.
209. Ibid.
210. National Archives, Collection of Alexander T. Augusta Letters.
211. Newby, *Anderson Ruffin Abbott*, 163.
212. Biographical Directory of the United States Congress, "Sumner, Charles." Charles Sumner was an antislavery senator from 1851 to 1874.
213. McPherson, *Ordeal by Fire*, 266. That law was passed in March 1865.
214. Quarles, *African American in the Civil War*, 204. "William Whiting, solicitor of the War Department, studied the Congressional Act of July 17, 1862, and concluded that persons of African descent were entitled to '$10 per month and one ration daily, of which monthly pay $3 per month may be in clothing.' At that time, white volunteers received $13 in cash, free uniforms, and full rations."
215. Newby, *Anderson Ruffin Abbott*, 80.
216. Agusta, "A.T. Augusta to the Editor of the Republican."
217. National Archives Record Group 94, A.R. Abbott Medical File.
218. Ibid.
219. Buxton Museum, "Jerome R. Riley."
220. Cobb, "A Short History of Freedmen's Hospital."
221. National Archives Record Group 94, A.R. Abbott Medical File.
222. Newby, *Anderson Ruffin Abbott*, 44.
223. Ibid., 47.
224. Ibid., 68–69. Referencing "Colored Female Corporate" in the *Messenger*.
225. National Parks Service, "United States Colored Troops."
226. Newby, *Anderson Ruffin Abbott*, 65.
227. Haskins, *Black Stars of Civil War Times*, 18.

228. McPherson, *Struggle for Equality*, 219.
229. Redkey, "Henry McNeal Turner: Black Chaplain in the Union Army."
230. Ibid.
231. Schultz, *Women at the Front*, 118.
232. Murphy, *Sojourner Truth*, 88.
233. Ibid., 93–94.
234. E.D.W.W. "Within These Walls."
235. Ibid.
236. Schultz, *Women at the Front*, 153.
237. E.D.W.W. "Within These Walls."
238. Record Group 94, Entry 578; Book 578 of Virginia Military Field Records of Hospitals, 1821–1912, Entry 544 in Record Group 94, Records of the Office of the Adjutant General, National Archives and Records Administration.
239. Friends of the Freedmen's Cemetery, "A House Divided Still Stands."
240. Drury, "Called to Arms in Civil War."
241. Ibid.
242. United States National Library of Medicine, "Binding Wounds."
243. Ibid.
244. Newby, *Anderson Ruffin Abbott*, 63.
245. Ibid.

Chapter 4

246. Ford, "Suffering in Silence."
247. Mapp, "Civil War: The Origins of Veterans' Health Care."
248. Maclean, "Cornelia Hancock."
249. Baldino, *Soldier's Friend*, 46.

Chapter 5

250. Cabiao, "Ray, Charlotte E." Of note, there were many successful African Americans in other fields in the Washington, D.C. area. Charlotte Ray is a good example. Born on January 13, 1850, in New York City, she would go on to be the first African American woman to practice law in the United States. Her parents moved to Washington, D.C., and she was educated at the Institution for the Education of Colored Youth. She graduated in 1869 and secretly applied to Howard Law School under the name C.E. Ray. She graduated in 1872 and was admitted to the D.C. bar on April 23, 1872. She

practiced in D.C. until 1879, when upon finding it too difficult to sustain her practice, she moved back to New York City.

251. Butts, "Alexander Thomas Augusta: Physician, Teacher and Human Rights Activist," 108.

252. "Purvis, Charles Burleigh (1842–1929)." The fight to integrate the local white medical society continued for many years; eventually the local society revised its regulations and allowed consultations with African American physicians.

253. Baker, Washington, Olakanmi, Savitt, Jacobs, Hoover and Wynia, "African American Physicians and Organized Medicine, 1846–1968."

254. "Purvis, Charles Burleigh (1842–1929)."

255. Angell, *Bishop Henry McNeal Turner*, 241–46.

256. Ibid.

257. Muller, *Frederick Douglass in Washigton, D.C.*, 77.

258. Peters, *Arlington National Cemetery*, 126. In a sad turn of fate, Robert Todd Lincoln was at or near the assasinations of Presidents Lincoln, Garfield and McKinley (who invited Robert Todd Lincoln to the Pan-American Exposition in Buffalo, New York, where he was shot by Leon Czolgosz on September 6, 1901). In later years, when asked about this and future presidential invitations to events, he replied, "No, I'm not going, and they'd better not ask me because there is a certain fatality about presidential function when I am present."

259. Ibid.

260. Butts, "Alexander Thomas Augusta: Physician, Teacher and Human Rights Activist," 108.

261. Howard University Archives Net, "Ex-Military Leaders." Dr. Augusta taught "Practical Anatomy," "Descriptive and Surgical Anatomy" and "Descriptive Microscopial and Surgical Anatomy." He was also a "Clinical Lecturer on Diseases of the Skin."

262. *Researching African American History at the National Archives: the Dr. Alexander T. Augusta Workshop*. "Even as an accomplished professor of medicine, Dr. Augusta encountered discrimination when he was denied acceptance to both the Medical Society of Washington, DC and the American Medical Association (AMA). Consequently, he and a protégé formed the National Medical Association (NMA). Unlike the AMA, the NMA had a nondiscriminatory membership policy."

263. United States National Library of Medicine. "Arlington National Cemetery."

264. Newby, *Anderson Ruffin Abbott*, 121–23.

265. Wilson, "Prejudice and Policy," S56.
266. Newmark, "Face to Face with History."
267. Taylor, *Reminiscences of My Life*, 55.
268. King, "In Search of Women of African Descent," 308.
269. Ibid.
270. Ibid.
271. Wikipedia, "Washington Afro American."
272. Wikipedia, "Washington Bee."
273. HarrietTubman.com, "Harriet Tubman: Civil War Pension."
274. Butts, "Alexander Thomas Augusta: Physician, Teacher and Human Rights Activist," 108.

EPILOGUE

275. Steckel, "A Peculiar Population" 722–41.
276. Newby, *Anderson Ruffin Abbott*, 61.
277. Bollet, "Analysis of the Medical Problems of the Civil War," 137.
278. Newby, *Anderson Ruffin Abbott*, 165.
279. Wilson, "Prejudice and Policy," S56.

Bibliography

Abdy, E.S. "Journal of a Residence and Tour in the United States of North America from April 1833 to October 1834." Vol. 2. London: John Murray. 1635. https://archive.org/stream/cihm_28465#page/n7/mode/2up.

Adams, George Worthington. *Doctors in Blue: The Medical History of the Union Army in the Civil War*. New York: H. Schuman, 1952.

African American Registry. "Alexander Augusta: A Pioneering Doctor." *African American Registry*. http://www.aaregistry.org/historic_events/view/alexander-augusta-pioneering-doctor.

Alcott, Louisa May. *Hospital Sketches*. Boston: James Redpath, 1863.

Angell, Stephen Ward. *Bishop Henry McNeal Turner and African-American Religion in the South*. Knoxville: University of Tennessee Press, 1992.

Aptheker, Herbert. "Negro Casualties in the Civil War." *Journal of Negro History* 32 (1947): 10–80.

Augusta, Alexander. "A.T. Augusta to the Editor of the Republican, 15 May 1863." *Christian Recorder*, May 30, 1863.

———. "Augusta to Captain C.W. Clippington, February 1, 1864." Printed in *Congressional Globe*, 265.

Baker, Robert, Harriet A. Washington, Ololade Olakanmi, Todd L. Savitt, Elizabeth A. Jacobs, Eddie Hoover and Matthew K. Wynia. "African American Physicians and Organized Medicine, 1846–1968: Origins of a Racial Divide." *Journal of the American Medical Association* (2008): 306–13.

Baldino, Georgiann. *A Soldier's Friend: Civil War Nurse Cornelia Hancock.* Naperville, IL: Pearl Editions, 2012.

Bayne-Jones, Stanhope. *The Evolution of Preventative Medicine in the United States Army, 1607–1939.* Washington, D.C.: Office of the Surgeon General Department of the Army, 1958.

Benson, Doug. "The Role of Chaplains in the Civil War." http://voices.yahoo.co/the-role-chaplains-civil-war-8472413.html.

Berlin, Ira, and Barbara Fields, eds. *Free at Last: A Documentary History of the Civil War.* Edison, NJ: Blue and Gray, 1997.

Berlin, Ira, Joseph Reidy and Leslia Rowland. *Freedom: A Documentary History of Emancipation.* Cambridge, UK: Cambridge University Press, 2010.

Biographical Directory of the United States Congress. "Sumner, Charles." http://bioguide.congress.gov/scripts/biodisplay.pl?index=S001068.

Black, Andrew K. "In the Service of the United States: Comparative Mortality Among African-American and White Troops in the Union Army." *Journal of Negro History* 79, no. 4 (1994): 317–33.

Bollet, Alfred Jay. "An Analysis of the Medical Problems of the Civil War." *Transactions of the American Clinical and Climatological Association* 103 (1992): 128–41.

Briggs, Walter De Blois. *Charles Edward Briggs: Civil War Surgeon in a Colored Regiment.* N.p., 1901.

Brinton, John H. *Personal Memoirs of John H. Brinton Major and Surgeon U.S.V. 1861–1865.* New York: Neale, 1914.

Brown, E. Richard. *Rockefeller Medicine Men: Medicine and Capitalism in America.* Los Angeles: University of California Press, 1981.

Burchard, Peter. *One Gallant Rush: Robert Gould Shaw and His Brave Black Regiment.* New York: St. Martin's Press, 1965.

Butts, Heather M. "Alexander Thomas Augusta: Physician, Teacher and Human Rights Activist." *Journal of the National Medical Association* 97, no. 1 (2005): 106–09.

Buxton Museum. "Jerome R. Riley." http://www.buxtonmuseum.com/history/PEOPLE/riley-jerome.html.

Byrd, W. Michael, and Linda A. Clayton. *An American Health Dilemma: A Medical History of African Americans and the Problem of Race: Beginnings to 1900.* New York: Routledge, 2000.

Cabiao, Howard. "Ray, Charlotte E. (1850–1911)." Blackpast.org. www.blackpast.org/aah/ray-charlotte-e-1850-1911.

Catton, Bruce, and Richard M. Ketchum. *The American Heritage Picture History of the Civil War.* New York: American Heritage, 1960.

Cobb, W.M. "Alexander Thomas Augusta, 1825–1890." *Journal of the National Medical Association* 44 (1952): 327–329.

———. "Nathan Frances Mossell, M.D., 1856–1946." *Journal of the National Medical Association* 46, no. 2 (1954): 118–130.

Crewe, Sandra Edmonds. "Harriet Tubman's Last Work: The Harriet Tubman Home for Aged and Indigent Negroes." *Journal of Gerontological Social Work* (2007): 229–44.

Cunningham, H.H. *Doctors in Gray*. Baton Rouge: Louisiana State University Press, 1958.

Delany, Martin R. *Blake; or, The Huts of America: a Novel.* Boston: Beacon Press, 1970.

———. *The Condition, Elevation, Emigration and Destiny of the Colored People of the United States*. New York: Arno Press, 1852.

———. *Principia of Ethnology: The Origin of Races and Color*. Philadelphia: Harper and Brother, 1879.

Dobak, William A. *Freedom by the Sword: The U.S. Colored Troops, 1862–1867*. Washington, D.C.: Center of Military History, 2011.

Drury, David. "Called to Arms in Civil War: Connecticut's Black Soldiers Respond." *Hartford Courant*, January 18, 2014. http://articles.courant.com/2014-01-18/news/hc-civil-war-black-troops-0119-20140118_1_colored-troops-william-webb-connecticut-volunteer-infantry.

Duncan, Russell, ed. *Blue-Eyed Child of Fortune: The Civil War Letters of Colonel Robert Gould Shaw*. Athens: University of Georgia Press, 1999.

EDWW. "Within These Walls: The Contraband Hospital and the African Americans Who Served There Feb 1st–28th; Opening Feb 10th 2010." Flickr. https://www.flickr.com/photos/esteemedhelga/4324822535/in/photostream/.

Emancipation Day. "Ending Slavery in the District of Columbia." District of Columbia. Emancipation.dc.gov/page/ending-slavery-district-columbia.

Emilio, Luis F. *A Brave Black Regiment: The History of the Fifty-fourth Regiment of Massachusetts Volunteer Infantry, 1863–1865*. New York: Da Capo, 1894.

Flannery, Michael. *Civil War Pharmacy: A History of Drugs, Drug Supply and Provision, and Therapeutics for the Union and Confederacy*. London: Informa Healthcare, 2004.

Fogel, Robert William, and Stanley L. Engerman. *Time on the Cross: The Economics of American Negro Slavery*. Boston: Little, Brown, 1974.

Ford, Sarah A.M. "Suffering in Silence: Psychological Disorders and Soldiers in the American Civil War." Armstrong State University. http://www.armstrong.edu/Initiatives/history_journal/history_journal_suffering_in_silence_psychological_disorders_and_soldiers_i.

Friends of the Freedmen's Cemetery. "A House Divided Still Stands: The Contraband Hospital and Alexandria Freedmen's Aid Workers." http://www.freedmenscemetery.org/resources/documents/contrabandhospital.pdf.

Garrison, W.B. *Civil War Curiosities: Strange Stories, Oddities, Events, and Coincidences*. Nashville, TN: Rutledge Hill, 1994.

Gates, Henry Louis, Jr., ed. *The Classic Slave Narratives*. Penguin Books, 2012.

Glatthaar, Joseph T. *Forged in Battle: The Civil War Alliance of Black Soldiers and White Officers*. Baton Rouge: Louisiana State University Press, 2009.

———. "'*Glory*,' the 54th Massachusetts Infantry, and Black Soldiers in the Civil War." *History Teacher* 24, no. 4 (August 1991): 475–85.

Gooding, James Henry. *On the Altar of Freedom: A Black Soldier's Civil War Letters from the Front*. Edited by Virginia M. Adams. Amherst: University of Massachusetts Press, 1991.

Greene, R.E. *African American Defenders of America, 1775–1973*. Chicago: Johnson, 1974.

Griffiths, D.L. "Medicine and Surgery in the American Civil War." *Proceedings of the Royal Society of Medicine* 59 (1966): 204–208.

HarrietTubman.com. "Harriet Tubman: Civil War Pension." http://harriettubman.com/pension.html.

Harris, Joseph Dennis. *A Summer on the Borders of the Caribbean Sea*. New York: A.B. Burdick, 1860.

Harrison, Robert. *Washington during the Civil War and Reconstruction: Race and Radicalism*. Cambridge, UK: Cambridge University Press, 2011.

Haskins, Jim, ed. *Black Stars of Civil War Times*. Hoboken, NJ: John Wiley and Sons, 2002.

Haviland, Laura S. *A Woman's Life-work: Labors and Experiences of Laura S. Haviland*. Cincinnati, OH: Walden and Stowe, 1882.

Hendrick, George, and Willene Hendrick. *Black Refugees in Canada: Accounts of Escape during the Era of Slavery*. Jefferson, NC: McFarland, 2010.

Howard University Archives Net. "Ex-Military Leaders." http://www.huarchivesnet.howard.edu/0008huarnet/muse2.htm.

Humez, Jean M. *The Life and the Life Stories of Harriet Tubman*. Madison: University of Wisconsin Press, 2005.

Humphreys, Margaret. *Intensely Human: The Health of the Black Soldier in the American Civil War*. Baltimore, MD: Johns Hopkins University Press, 2008.

Hunter, Jeanne. "For Freed Blacks in the Civil War, Washington Was a City of Contradictions." *Washington Post*, October 7, 2011.

Kass, Amalie M. "Dr. Thomas Hodgkin, Dr. Martin Delany, and the Return to Africa." *Medical History* (1983): 374–75.

Kaufman, Howard H. "Treatment of Head Injuries in the American Civil War." *Journal of Neurosurgery* 78 (1993): 838–45.

King, Lisa Y. "In Search of Women of African Descent Who Served in the Civil War Union Navy." *Journal of Negro History* 83, no. 4 (Autumn 1998): 302–09.

Lamb, D.S. *A Historical, Biographical and Statistical Souvenir*. Washington, D.C.: Medical Faculty of Howard University, 1900.

Lee, Chulhee. "Socioeconomic Differences in the Health of Black Union Army Soldiers." *Social Science History* 33 (2009): 427–57.

Levine, Robert S., ed. *Martin R. Delany: A Documentary Reader*. Chapel Hill: University of North Carolina Press, 2003.

Lincoln, Abraham. "Letter to Horace Greeley." Abraham Lincoln Online. http://www.abrahamlincolnonline.org/lincoln/speeches/greeley.htm.

Lowe, Tony B. "Nineteenth Century Review of Mental Healthcare for African Americans: A Legacy of Service and Policy Barriers." *Journal of Sociology and Social Welfare* 33, no. 4 (2006): 29–50.

MacDonald, John. *Historical Atlas of the Civil War*. Edison, NJ: Chartwell Books, 2010.

Maclean, Maggie. "Cornelia Hancock." Civil War Women. http://civilwarwomenblog.com/cornelia-hancock/.

Mapp, Jerome W. "The Civil War: The Origins of Veterans' Health Care." United States Department of Veterans Affairs. http://www.va.gov/health/NewsFeatures/20110413a.asp.

Margo, Robert A., and Richard H. Steckel. "The Heights of American Slaves: New Evidence on Slave Nutrition and Health." *Social Science History* 6 (1982): 516–38.

McPherson, James M. *The Negro's Civil War: How American Blacks Felt and Acted During the War for the Union*. New York: Ballantine Books, 1965.

———. *Ordeal by Fire: The Civil War and Reconstruction*. 2nd ed. New York: McGraw-Hill, 1992.

———. *The Struggle for Equality: Abolitionists and the Negro in the Civil War and Reconstruction*. 2nd ed. Princeton, NJ: Princeton University Press, 1967.

Morais, Herbert M. *The History of the Afro-American in Medicine*. Cornwells Heights, PA: Publishers Agency, 1978.

Mossell, Nathan Frances. "Autobiography." University of Pennsylvania Archives. http://www.archives.upenn.edu/primdocs/upf/upf1_9ar/mossell_nf/mossell_nf_autobio.pdf.

Muller, John. *Frederick Douglass in Washington, D.C.: The Lion of Anacostia*. Charleston, SC: The History Press, 2012.

Murphy, Larry. *Sojourner Truth: A Biography*. Santa Barbara, CA: Greenwood Biographies, 2011.

National Archives. Collection of Alexander T. Augusta Letters. Washington, D.C.: National Archives and Records Administration.

———. Record Group 94. A.R. Abbott Medical File. Personal Papers of Medical Officers and Physicians Prior to 1912. Records of the Office of the Adjutant General. Washington, D.C.: National Archives and Records Administration.

———. Record Group 94. Virginia Military Field Records of Hospitals, 1821–1912. Records of the Office of the Adjutant General. Washington, D.C.: National Archives and Records Administration.

National Parks Service. "The United States Colored Troops and the Defenses of Washington." http://www.nps.gov/resources/story.htm?id=207.

Newby, M. Dalyce. *Anderson Ruffin Abbott: First Afro-Canadian Doctor*. Markham, ON: Associated Medical Services: Fitzhenry and Whiteside, 1998.

Newmark, Jill L. "Contraband Hospital, 1862–1863: Health Care for the First Freedpeople" Blackpast.org. http://www.blackpast.org/perspectives/contraband-hospital-1862-1863-health-care-first-freedpeople.

———. "Face to Face with History." National Archives. http://www.archives.gov/publications/prologue/2009/fall/face.html.

Oates, Stephen. *A Woman of Valor: Clara Barton and the Civil War*. New York: Free Press, 1994.

Painter, Nell Irvin. *Sojourner Truth: A Life, A Symbol*. New York: W.W. Norton: 1997.

Peters, James Edward. *Arlington National Cemetery: Shrine to America's Heroes*. 2nd ed. Bethesda, MD: Woodbine House, 2000.

Powers, Bernard Edward. *Black Charlestonians: A Social History, 1822–1885*. Fayetteville: University of Arkansas Press, 1999.

Price, James S. *The Battle of New Market Heights Freedom: Will Be Theirs by the Sword*. Charleston, SC: The History Press, 2011.

"Purvis, Charles Burleigh (1842–1929)—Surgeon, Physician, Educator, Chronology, Attends College and Joins the Military—Medical, Howard, Board, and University." Online Encyclopedia. http://encyclopedia.jrank.org/articles/pages/4428/Purvis.

Quarles, B. *The African American in the Civil War*. New York: De Capo, 1989.

Randolph, Lewis A. *Rights for a Season: Politics of Race, Class, and Gender in Richmond, Virginia*. Knoxville: University of Tennessee Press, 2003.

Redkey, Edwin S. "Black Chaplains in the Union Army." *Civil War History* 33, no. 4 (1987): 331–50.

———. "Henry McNeal Turner: Black Chaplain in the Union Army." in *Black Soldiers in Blue*. Edited by John David Smith. Chapel Hill: University of North Carolina Press, 2002.

Reid, Richard M., ed. *Practicing Medicine in a Black Regiment: The Civil War Diary of Burt G. Wilder, 55th Massachusetts*. Amherst: University of Massachusetts Press, 2010.

Researching African American History at the National Archives: The Dr. Alexander T. Augusta Workshop. Washington, D.C.: National Archives Tour Office, 1994. U.S. National Archives and Records Administration Services publication SuDoc AE 1.102:H 62/4.

Ruthow, Lainie W., and Ira M. Ruthow. "Homeopaths, Surgery and the Civil War: Edward C. Franklin and the Struggle to Achieve Medical Pluralism in the Union Army." *Archives of Surgery* 139 (2004): 785–791.

Sattelmeyer, Robert. "Miss Alcott Goes to War." *Civil War Times* 2, no. 51 (April 2012): 44.

Savitt, T. *Four African-American Proprietary Medical Colleges: 1888–1923*. London: Oxford University Press, 2000.

Schouler, William. *A History of Massachusetts in the Civil War*. Vol. 1. Boston: Dutton, 1868.

Schroeder-Lein, Glenna R. *The Encyclopedia of Civil War Medicine*. Armonk, NY: M.E. Sharpe, 2008.

Schultz, Jane E. *Women at the Front: Hospital Workers in Civil War America*. Chapel Hill: University of North Carolina Press, 2004.

Schwartz, Gerald, ed. *A Woman Doctor's Civil War: Esther Hill Hawk's Diary*. Columbia: University of South Carolina Press, 1989.

Simmons, William J., and Henry McNeal Turner. *Men of Mark: Eminent, Progressive and Rising*. Cleveland, OH: Geo. M. Rewell and Company, 1887.

Smith, John David, ed. *Black Soldiers in Blue: African American Troops in the Civil War Era*. Chapel Hill: University of North Carolina Press, 2003.

Sollors, Werner, Caldwell Titcomb, Thomas Underwood and Randall Kennedy. *Blacks at Harvard: A Documentary History of African-American Experience at Harvard and Radcliffe*. New York: New York University Press, 1993.

Sparks, Tanner. "James Slaughter." Archives of Maryland. http://msa.maryland.gov/megafile/msa/speccol/sc3500/sc3520/003700/003783/html/03783bio.html.

Steckel, Richard H. "A Peculiar Population: The Nutrition, Health and Mortality of American Slaves from Childhood to Maturity." *Journal of Economic History* 46 (1986): 721–41.

Steven. "The 1st U.S. Colored Troops at Roosevelt Island." Civil War Washington, D.C. http://civilwarwashingtondc1861-1865.blogspot.com/2012/02/1st-us-colored-troops-at-roosevelt.html.

Taylor, Susie King. *Reminiscences of My Life in Camp with the 33d United States Colored Troops Late 1st S.C. Volunteers*. Boston: self-published, 1902.

Thomson, Samuel. *New Guide to Health, or Botanic Family Physician*. Boston: E.G. House, 1822.

Tomblin, Barbara Brooks. *Bluejackets and Contrabands: African Americans and the Union Navy*. Lexington: University of Kentucky Press, 2009.

United States Census Bureau. "Census of Population and Housing." https://www.census.gov/prod/www/decennial.html.

———. "District of Columbia—Race and Hispanic Origin: 1800 to 1990." http://www.census.gov/population/www/documentation/twps0056/tab23.pdf.

United States National Library of Medicine. "Arlington National Cemetery." http://www.nlm.nih.gov/hmd/medtour/arlington.html.

———. "Binding Wounds, Pushing Boundaries: African Americans in Civil War Medicine." http://www.nlm.nih.gov/exhibition/bindingwounds/within.html.

Voices of the Civil War. "Christian Fleetwood." Library of Congress. http://blogs.loc.gov/civil-war-voices/about/christian-fleetwood/.

Waddell, Joseph Addison. *Annals of Augusta County, Virginia, from 1726 to 1871*. 2nd ed. Staunton, VA: C.R. Caldwell, 1902.

Whitman, Walt. *Leaves of Grass*. New York: Penguin, 1855.

Wikipedia. "Laura Smith Haviland." En.wikipedia.org/wiki/laura_smith_Haviland.

———. "Washington Afro American." En.wikipedia.org/wiki/The_Washington_Afro_American.

———. "Washington Bee." En.wikipedia.org/wiki/Washington_bee.

Wilson, Keith P. *Campfires of Freedom: The Camp Life of Black Soldiers during the Civil War*. Kent, OH: Kent State University Press, 2002.

Wilson, Sven E. "Prejudice and Policy: Racial Discrimination in the Union Army Disability Pension System, 1865–1906." *American Journal of Public Health* 100, Supplemental 1 (2010): S56–65.

Yacovone, Donald, ed. *A Voice of Thunder: The Civil War Letters of George E. Stephens*. Champaign: University of Illinois Press, 1997.

Zwierzyna, John. "Nicholas Biddle." 150 Pennsylvania Civil War. Pacivilwar150.com/throughpeople/AfricanAmericans/Nicholasbiddle.

INDEX

D

E

F

G

H

J

K

L

M

N

O

P

About the Author

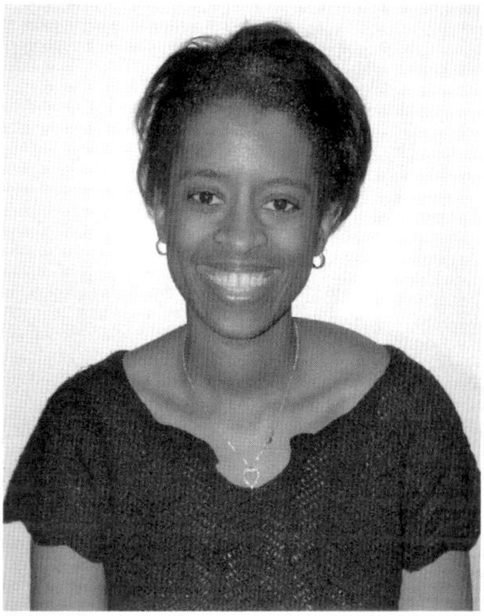

Heather Butts JD, MPH, MA, is an Integration of Science and Practice (ISP) instructor and faculty advisor of the Part-Time Health Policy Management students at Columbia University, Mailman School of Public Health, where she teaches bioethics and public health law. She also serves as an adjunct professor in health law and bioethics at Saint John's School of Law. She is the co-founder of HEALTH for Youths, Inc., which focusses on college readiness, outreach to underserved youth and community service. She is a board member for the nonprofit Northside Center for Child Development. She is also the founder of the online training and education company LEARN for Life Consulting, LLC, and does college readiness and preparation counseling for high school students.

She previously served as regulatory specialist at Columbia University Medical Center's Institutional Review Board and focused on compliance audits, training, education and privacy issues. Prior to her work at Columbia, Butts served as senior associate in the Healthcare Regulatory Group of Pricewaterhouse Coopers, LLP, where she focused on regulatory compliance issues.

Butts received her BA from Princeton University, her JD from Saint John's University School of Law, her MPH from Harvard University School of Public Health and her MA in education from Teachers College.

Her publications include *Alexander Thomas Augusta: Physician, Teacher and Human Rights Activist.*